Nurturing Life Within

The Essential Nutrition for Pregnancy and Expecting Mothers

By

Melissa W. Giblin

Nurturing Life Within

Copyright

Disclaimer

This book serves as informative support, not medical counsel. Melissa W. Giblin, the author, is not a medical professional. Readers are advised to consult medical professionals for tailored guidance. The content's general nature may not apply universally, and individual results may differ. Any specific medical procedures discussed are for informational purposes, not endorsements. While efforts ensure accuracy, the author disclaims responsibility for errors. Readers assume responsibility for their decisions and release the author from any claims arising from book use. Prioritize personal health; seek professional advice for personalized care.

Table of Content

Introduction

The Importance of Nutrition during Pregnancy

Your body goes through a series of astonishing modifications during the incredible journey of bringing new life into the world. Throughout this amazing process, the importance of nutrition during pregnancy emerges as a critical aspect that not only sustains the mother but also has a significant impact on the unborn child's growth and development.

Your body becomes a vehicle of life the minute you learn the joyful news of your upcoming parenthood. It is responsible for nourishing and sustaining the precious being growing within. Nutrition during pregnancy is more than just food; it is the foundation of a healthy and thriving journey for both you and your baby.

As you embark on this wonderful journey, it becomes clear that what you consume serves as the foundation for your baby's first home. Every bit of food has the power to mold your child's health foundation, influencing everything from cognitive development to overall well-being.

Your body experiences fast changes throughout the early stages of pregnancy in order to produce a supportive environment. Proper nutrition becomes critical because it provides the necessary nutrients for the production of critical structures such as the neural tube, which eventually develops into the brain and spinal cord. A delicate ballet of vitamins and minerals orchestrates a growth symphony, setting the groundwork for a healthy future.

Adequate nutrition is about more than simply providing basic needs; it's about creating the best environment for your baby to thrive. Folic acid, found in green leafy vegetables and legumes, is an important nutrient in avoiding neural tube abnormalities. You actively contribute to the delicate tapestry of your child's early development by eating these nutrient-rich foods.

Nutrition during pregnancy effects cognitive function and intellectual capacity, in addition to physical health. Omega-3 fatty acids are well-known for their involvement in brain development and can be found in fatty fish and flaxseeds. By including these in your baby's diet, you're creating a strong foundation for his or her cognitive talents, supporting a future of learning and exploration.

However, the necessity of nutrition extends beyond your growing baby's immediate demands. It protects your personal well-being, allowing you to face the challenges of pregnancy with strength and vitality. Adequate iron consumption avoids anemia, keeps your energy levels up, and supports the increased blood volume required for both you and the baby.

Nutrition has an impact on delivery outcomes and postnatal health even after the pregnancy has ended. A well-nourished body is better able to endure the demands of labor and recover quickly postpartum. The nutritional decisions you make become an investment in your family's overall health and energy.

Remember that balance is essential while you relish the broad assortment of foods that contribute to your well-being. Each vitamin has a specific purpose, and a diversified diet ensures that you get a wide range of critical elements. While cravings can take you on exciting gastronomic experiences, it is the combination of these sensations that adds to the complete nutrition essential for a successful pregnancy.

Consult with healthcare providers to adjust your diet to your specific needs while on this nutritious journey. Prenatal care is a collaborative effort, and your healthcare team may provide specialized guidance to ensure you get the correct mix of nutrients tailored to your specific needs.

To summarize, the significance of nutrition during pregnancy goes beyond the act of eating; it's a celebration of life, a purposeful decision to nurture and cherish the magnificent journey you're embarking on. As you cherish each bite, remember that you're not only feeding yourself, but also shaping the destiny of the beautiful life growing inside you. Accept the power of nutrition as a guiding factor as you traverse the incredible journey to motherhood.

The Role of Vitamins and Supplements

You will come across a composition of nutrients regulating an amazing masterpiece of life as you explore the undiscovered waters of pregnancy. Vitamins and supplements emerge as essential parts in this knowledgeable structure, each giving its own harmony to the growth of a healthy pregnancy.

The beginning of this symphony acknowledges the critical function that vitamins play in supporting life. Vitamins, which are classed as water-soluble or fat-soluble, are chemical molecules that your body requires in specific proportions for various physiological processes. Water-soluble vitamins, such as vitamin C and the B-complex vitamins, are like ephemeral dancers, gracefully gliding through your system, but fat-soluble vitamins, such as A, D, E, and K, find refuge in the lipid layers, weaving their spell over time.

When you enter the world of pregnancy, the need for these vitamins multiplies, producing a need that goes above and beyond the ordinary. Consider vitamin A, which protects embryonic growth. It is found in brilliant orange vegetables such as carrots and sweet potatoes and plays an important role in the development of your baby's eyes, skin, and internal organs. In this symphony of life, vitamin A takes center stage, creating the blueprint for your child's physical existence.

Meanwhile, the B-complex vitamins emerge as the flexible instrumentalists, contributing to a wide range of functions. Vitamin B6, found in bananas and avocados, aids in the development of your baby's brain and neurological system. Folate, a virtuoso in this ensemble, steps into the spotlight, preventing neural tube abnormalities and maintaining the smooth orchestration of cell division. Its sources, which range from lentils to leafy greens, become the notes that build the delicate melody of a healthy pregnancy.

Zooming out, vitamin C takes on the role of conductor, orchestrating a harmonic collagen production. It is found in citrus fruits and strawberries and helps to strengthen your baby's connective tissues, skin, and bones. As the symphony develops, vitamin D takes center stage, promoting calcium and phosphorus absorption for your baby's skeletal system development. This nutrient dances on the stage of sunlight, casting a bright influence on your path.

Further, vitamin E enhances the performance with its antioxidant properties. This vitamin protects your developing baby's cells from oxidative stress by passing through nuts, seeds, and spinach. The fat-soluble ballet continues with vitamin K, which orchestrates the delicate dance of blood clotting, protecting both you and your baby from potential threats.

The vitamins create a symphony of perfect health by fluidly transitioning between these fat-soluble and water-soluble activities, setting the groundwork for the flourishing life within you. Balance, however, is essential in this delicate dance. Any of these vitamins, in excess or shortage, can upset the delicate balance, emphasizing the significance of a well-rounded and diverse diet.

As the symphony continues, supplements enter the stage as supporting players, providing assistance when food sources fall short. Prenatal vitamins, like a thorough musical score, embody a spectrum of critical nutrients adapted to the special demands of pregnancy. These supplements act as a safety net, ensuring that your body receives the nutrients it requires even when your diet is limited.

Folic acid's importance in the supplement world is once again highlighted. It is a synthetic type of folate that plays an important function in avoiding neural tube abnormalities during the critical early stages of pregnancy. Folic acid supplements become a trustworthy partner in the broad tapestry of your nutritional journey, reinforcing the foundation created by dietary sources.

Omega-3 fatty acids, another significant supplement player, carve a special place in the performance. These nutrients, which are rich in fatty fish and flaxseeds, aid in the development of your baby's brain and eyes. They transit the various paths of your circulatory system, enriching the makeup of cell membranes and sustaining the colorful crescendo of life.

The supplementary landscape also includes iron, which is required for hemoglobin production. Iron supplements become a steadfast ally while your body experiences the magnificent change of making more blood to support your growing baby, preventing anemia and guaranteeing the smooth flow of oxygen to both you and your child.

Calcium supplements, which are essential for bone and tooth fortification, appear as protagonists in the supplement narrative. While dairy products and leafy greens add to your calcium intake, supplements stand ready to reinforce this crucial element, establishing the basis for your baby's future skeletal symphony.

However, the supplement journey is not without complexities. As with any performance, interaction with healthcare specialists serves as the guiding conductor, adapting the composition to your specific needs. The dosage, timing, and specific supplements are determined by a number of factors, including your overall health, dietary habits, and pregnancy-specific requirements.

The overall concept of vitamins and supplements remains one of harmony and balance. Your body, as a receptacle of life, becomes the stage for this symphony to unfold. The notes of each vitamin and supplement resound, influencing your child's destiny and boosting your own well-being.

Chapter 1

Nutritional Foundations in Pregnancy

Essential Nutrients for a Healthy Pregnancy

You find yourself engaged in a world where every word has the ability to change not only the state of your health but the future of the life developing within as you embark on the awe-inspiring journey of pregnancy. Let's look at the nutritional foundations of a healthy pregnancy in this chapter, an opportunity filled with the essential nutrients that weave an intricate tapestry of growth and vitality for both you and your baby.

1. Protein: The Builder of Growth

Protein develops as a crucial pillar, the architect of cellular building, once one enters the realm of pregnancy. Proteins are the fundamental building blocks of life, and they play an important part in the development of your baby's organs, tissues, and muscles. Lean meats, poultry, fish, eggs, dairy, beans, and legumes become the artistic strokes on this protein canvas, guaranteeing that life unfolds with resilience and strength.

2. Calcium: Bone Health and Beyond

Consider calcium to be the mortar that strengthens your baby's bones and teeth. As your baby's skeletal system develops, sources including dairy products, leafy greens, and fortified foods become reservoirs of this important mineral. Ensuring a sufficient calcium intake not only helps your baby's growth but also protects your own bone health when pregnant.

3. Iron: The Oxygen Conductor

Iron acts as a conductor in this life symphony, managing the supply of oxygen to both you and your developing kid. As your blood volume expands during pregnancy, iron-rich foods such as lean meats, fortified cereals, and dark leafy greens become the tools that help this critical process run smoothly. Iron helps your baby's developing cells obtain the oxygen they require, contributing to a robust and healthy trip.

4. Folate: Neural Landscape Nurturing

The influence of folate, a B-vitamin with the ability to prevent neural tube abnormalities, shapes the landscape of neural development. The brushstrokes that pour this vitamin into your nutritional canvas are dark leafy greens, legumes, citrus fruits, and fortified cereals. Folate is not only an ally in the avoidance of birth abnormalities, but it also plays an active role in the orchestration of DNA synthesis, emphasizing its relevance in the life design.

5. Omega-3 Fatty Acids: Brain and Eye Nutrition

Welcome to the world of omega-3 fatty acids, the protectors of cognitive growth and visual acuity. Fatty fish, flaxseeds, chia seeds, and walnuts act as carriers for these necessary fats in your diet. Omega-3 fatty acids help your baby's brain and eyes develop, laying the framework for a future filled with curiosity and visual exploration.

6. Vitamin D: The Sunshine Vitamin

Consider vitamin D to be the radiance of the sun, influencing calcium and phosphorus absorption. As your baby's skeletal system develops, exposure to sunlight and dietary sources such as fatty fish and fortified dairy products provide avenues for vitamin D to contribute to the formation of strong and healthy bones.

7. Collagen Composer (Vitamin C)

Vitamin C acts as a composer in the symphony of collagen production, orchestrating the formation of connective tissues, skin, and bones. Citrus fruits, strawberries, bell peppers, and broccoli serve as vehicles for incorporating this vitamin into your diet. Vitamin C not only benefits your own tissue health, but it also helps to build a strong foundation for your baby's growth.

8. Zinc: The Cellular Designer

When we zoom in on the microscopic level, zinc emerges as the cellular architect, affecting cell division and proliferation. Zinc, which may be found in meat, dairy, nuts, and whole grains, becomes the elemental power that ensures your baby's cells grow and thrive. This essential mineral emerges as an unsung hero in the story of cellular formation, providing the framework for life's complicated dance.

9. Vitamin A: Visionary Nutrition

Vitamin A provides the visionary sustenance for both you and your kid in the tapestry of vision and immune function. Vitamin A, which is found in bright vegetables such as carrots, sweet potatoes, and spinach, aids in the development of your baby's eyes, skin, and immune system. The rich colors of these foods serve as a palette for this crucial vitamin to find its place in your nutritious artwork.

10. Vitamin E: Antioxidant Protector

As the symphony of life develops, vitamin E takes the stage as the antioxidant guardian, protecting your and your baby's cells from oxidative stress. Nuts, seeds, spinach, and broccoli serve as conduits for this vitamin to bring vigor into your diet. Vitamin E guarantees that the delicate dance of cell formation takes place in an environment free of oxidative damage.

11. Magnesium for Muscular Harmony

Magnesium, known as the "Maestro of Muscular Harmony," has an impact on muscle function and nerve transmission. Whole grains, nuts, and leafy greens become the routes through which magnesium contributes to the preservation of a healthy musculoskeletal system as your body undergoes the extraordinary change of pregnancy. It transforms into a silent power that supports your physical journey while also safeguarding your baby's well-being.

12. Hydration: Keeping the Canvas Fluid

Hydration appears as the silent yet crucial artist among the multitude of nutrients, supporting the fluid canvas of your body. Water serves as a conduit for nutrients to be transported, waste to be expelled, and the amniotic fluid wrapping your baby to thrive. Maintaining appropriate hydration becomes a vital element as you advance through the stages of pregnancy, enabling the smooth continuation of this remarkable journey.

These vital nutrients converge in the magnificent tapestry of a healthy pregnancy, each performing a different yet interwoven part in the symphony of life. Protein, calcium, iron, folate, omega-3 fatty acids, vitamin D, vitamin C, zinc, vitamin A, vitamin E, magnesium, and water work together to create a vivid composition that promises a flourishing and robust journey for both you and your kid.

Balanced Diet for Expectant Mothers

The Macronutrient Canvas: A Well-Balanced Palette

Imagine a canvas rich in macronutrients—carbohydrates, proteins, and fats—as you enter the domain of a balanced diet for pregnancy. Carbohydrates, the energy fuel, are derived from whole grains, fruits, and vegetables and provide a consistent energy release that is required for the dynamic changes that your body goes through. Protein, the architect of growth, may be found in lean meats, poultry, fish, beans, and legumes, and it helps your baby's organs and tissues develop. Avocados, almonds, seeds, and olive oil provide the brushstrokes that enrich the canvas, aiding cellular development and ensuring a well-rounded foundation.

The Micronutrient Mosaic: Essential Elements

Micronutrients emerge as the important pieces that adorn the canvas of a balanced diet when we zoom into the intricate intricacies of the mosaic. Consider a color palette in which each color represents a different nutrient—vitamins and minerals that are carefully woven into the fabric of your regular meals. Dark leafy greens are transformed into emerald strokes of folate, a B-vitamin that is essential for neural development. Orange vegetables, such as carrots and sweet potatoes, contain vitamin A pigments that promote vision and immunological function.

Nuts and seeds, which resemble bronze and gold, provide zinc and vitamin E, serving as antioxidants and promoting cellular harmony. Berries' vivid blues and purples indicate the presence of vitamin C and antioxidants, which strengthen your immune system and aid in collagen creation. Meanwhile, calcium-rich whites from dairy products and fortified diets help to build strong bones and teeth.

Fluids: Life's Sustaining Waters

Imagine a continual flow—the sustaining streams of life—amid the brilliant colors and textures. Hydration transforms into a flowing brush, permeating every area of the canvas. Water, herbal teas, and fresh fruit juices help meet fluid requirements for nutrient transfer, waste disposal, and the amniotic fluid that surrounds your baby. Adequate hydration improves digestion and ensures a buoyant environment for your baby's development by supporting dynamic changes in blood volume.

Portioning: Achieving Balance in Quantity and Quality

Consider the principle of portioning to be the balancing factor in this artistic production. During pregnancy, your body's dietary needs change, and portion restriction becomes the governing concept. A balanced diet entails spreading out your meals throughout the day to provide a consistent supply of nutrients. Small, regular meals help to minimize nausea and optimize nutrient absorption.

Imagine a plate divided into pieces as you plan your meals: half packed with bright vegetables and fruits, a quarter with lean proteins, and a quarter with complete grains. This visual signal acts as a practical guidance, providing a diverse nutrient intake. Make each meal a celebration of nourishment by incorporating a range of food colors, textures, and flavors to improve the sensory experience.

Supplemental Materials: Bridging the Gaps
Supplements appear as bridging items that cover potential gaps in the nuanced composition of a healthy diet for pregnant moms. While whole foods establish the groundwork, prenatal vitamins act as a safety net, ensuring that your body receives necessary nutrients even if your diet is limited. These supplements frequently contain folic acid, iron, calcium, vitamin D, and omega-3 fatty acids, providing a complete approach to supporting the particular demands of pregnancy.

Mindful Eating: Developing Awareness

Consider mindful eating to be the meditative brushstroke that cultivates awareness in the wide landscape of a balanced diet. Savoring each bite, paying attention to hunger and fullness cues, and enjoying the sensory experience of food are all part of mindful eating. Engage your senses by observing the colors, textures, and scents of your food. Chew slowly to allow digestion to begin in the mouth. Mindfulness practice at meals promotes a connection with the nourishing qualities of food, promoting a positive relationship with your dietary choices.

Culinary Exploration: A Flavor Journey

Imagine culinary exploration as an adventurous trip of flavors as you navigate the terrain of a balanced diet. Accept a wide range of cuisines, experiment with herbs and spices, and learn about the rich fabric of global culinary traditions. This research not only improves the palatability of your meals, but it also broadens the range of nutrients your body obtains. The world of food transforms into a bright palette, delivering a plethora of flavors that add to the complexity and depth of your nutritional journey.

Intuitive Gastronomy: Listening to Cravings

Cravings become the instinctive gastronomical notes that your body orchestrates on this culinary voyage. Pay attention to these cues—cravings frequently convey messages about specific dietary requirements. While satisfying appetites, maintain balance by including nutrient-dense foods. Do you have a sweet tooth? Choose fruits. Do you want anything savory? Select whole-grain snacks. Trusting your body's messages strengthens your symbiotic relationship with your nutritional requirements, promoting a sense of connection and harmony.

Warnings and Recommendations: Navigating Dietary Challenges

Be aware of cautions and considerations within the broad canvas of a balanced diet. Certain meals can be dangerous during pregnancy, and understanding these nuances is critical for a safe and successful journey. Raw seafood, unpasteurized dairy, excessive caffeine, and certain types of fish with high mercury concentration all necessitate caution. Consult with a healthcare practitioner to help you manage these dietary obstacles, and make sure your culinary choices are in line with the health of both you and your kid.

Culinary Pleasure: A Joyful Feast

Finally, imagine food delight as a joyous feast that pervades your nutritional journey. Accept the enjoyment of food, enjoy the flavors, and enjoy the sensation of sustaining your body and the life within. Cultivating a positive relationship with food improves the emotional and psychological aspects of your pregnancy, providing a joyful and satisfying atmosphere.

Recognize that this culinary symphony is a dynamic and evolving composition as you immerse yourself in the preparation of a balanced diet for pregnant mothers. The needs of your body alter with each trimester, and modifying your nutritional choices accordingly allows a smooth passage through the wonderful phases of pregnancy. Accept the nutritional palette, relish the tastes, and let the painting of your balanced diet be a monument to the artistry of nourishing life.

Chapter 2

The Key Vitamins During Pregnancy

Vitamin A: Promoting Growth and Vision

Imagine Vitamin A as a guardian, watching over the complicated processes of growth and vision as you investigate its role in pregnancy. Vitamin A is well-known for its involvement in the development of your baby's numerous organs and tissues. It is especially important in promoting the development of the heart, lungs, kidneys, eyes, and bones during the early stages of pregnancy, when these foundational structures are taking shape.

One of Vitamin A's key tasks is to influence vision. Vitamin A is required by the retina, a light-sensitive layer at the back of the eye, to make pigments required for low-light and color vision. The delicate dance of photoreceptor cells, aided by Vitamin A, ensures that your baby's eyes develop properly for visual acuity.

Aside from these fundamental functions, Vitamin A protects the immune system. It helps to create and maintain healthy skin and mucous membranes, which are the body's first line of defense against infections. As your pregnancy progresses, ensuring a sufficient intake of Vitamin A becomes increasingly important in bolstering both your own and your baby's immune resilience.

Vitamin A Sources: A Colorful Palette of Nutrients

Consider a colorful pallet on your plate, with each hue reflecting a high source of Vitamin A. Explore the vast assortment of foods that provide an abundance of Vitamin A in various forms as you strive to incorporate this critical component into your diet.

Beta-Carotene: Nature's Vitamin A Precursor
Explore the world of beta-carotene, a provitamin A molecule found in a variety of bright fruits and vegetables. Carrots, sweet potatoes, spinach, kale, mangoes, and cantaloupes are high in beta-carotene, which acts as a precursor to vitamin A in nature. These plant-based molecules are converted into active Vitamin A by the body as needed, providing a regulated and safe dose of this critical nutrient.

Animal Sources of Retinol: Meats and Dairy
Include animal-based sources of Vitamin A, where the substance is found in its active form, retinol. Retinol is widely available in liver, fish, eggs, and dairy products such as milk and cheese, which contributes to overall Vitamin A intake. While these sources are effective, it's important to balance your intake because too much retinol can be harmful during pregnancy.

Nutrient-Rich Ecosystem: Leafy Greens

Consider leafy greens to be a nutrient-rich environment that contains a variety of vitamins and minerals, including Vitamin A. Spinach, kale, collard greens, and Swiss chard provide beta-carotene to your diet, increasing not only Vitamin A intake but also a plethora of other critical elements necessary for a healthy pregnancy.

Nature's Desserts: Brightly Colored Fruits

As you enjoy nature's desserts—brightly colored fruits—relax knowing that you're also providing your body with Vitamin A. Vibrant fruits and vegetables such as papaya, apricots, mangoes, and watermelon provide a wonderful method to achieve your nutrient requirements while also adding taste and health benefits to your diet.

Root Vegetables: Natural Nutritional The riches

Root vegetables, like earthy nutritional jewels, contribute to your Vitamin A consumption. Sweet potatoes, carrots, and butternut squash not only provide flavor to your meals, but they also provide beta-carotene to your body, providing a harmonious balance in your vitamin profile.

How to Balance Vitamin A Intake During Pregnancy

It's critical to establish a balance when incorporating vitamin A-rich foods into your diet. Excessive intake of vitamin A, particularly retinol from animal sources, may offer concerns during pregnancy. High doses of retinol have been linked to birth abnormalities, making it critical to monitor your overall consumption.

Adopt a multifaceted approach, combining beta-carotene-rich plant sources with moderate amounts of animal-based choices. This not only assures a safer consumption, but also a broader spectrum of nutrients necessary for a healthy pregnancy.

Consult with your healthcare provider to adjust your Vitamin A consumption to your specific needs. They can offer advice based on your overall health, dietary habits, and special pregnancy-related needs.

Finally, Vitamin A is Beneficial to Life

Allow Vitamin A to be your ally as you navigate the seas of nutrition during pregnancy—a guardian nourishing the growth and vision of your precious creation. Accept the rainbow of hues on your plate, relishing the broad range of foods that contribute to a healthy and enriching diet.

Vitamin A plays an important role in the great story of pregnancy, contributing to the fragile symphony of life within you. You can harness the benefits of this crucial vitamin with a conscious and balanced approach, ensuring a harmonious journey toward a healthy and vibrant motherhood.

Vitamin B-Complex: B6, B12, and folate

You find yourself engrossed in the delicate dance of critical nutrients that shape the bright tapestry of life within as you embark on the extraordinary journey of pregnancy. In this chapter, we'll look at the Vitamin B-complex, which is a group of three B-vitamins: B6, B12, and folate. They collaborate to create a symphony of cellular operations that are critical for the development and well-being of both you and your growing kid.

Vitamin B6: Metabolic Mastermind

Consider Vitamin B6 to be the metabolic maestro who maintains a harmonious equilibrium within your body. This water-soluble vitamin, commonly known as pyridoxine, is essential during pregnancy for a variety of physiological activities.

1. Amino Acid Metabolism: Cellular Building Block Nurturing

Consider amino acids to be the building blocks of life, and Vitamin B6 to be the nurturing force that aids in their metabolism. Vitamin B6 promotes the synthesis and breakdown of amino acids during pregnancy, when cellular growth is at its highest, promoting the development of tissues, muscles, and organs in both you and your baby.

2. Neurotransmitter Production: Mood and Cognitive Balancing

Consider Vitamin B6 to be a regulator of neurotransmitters, which are chemical messengers that influence mood and cognition. This vitamin helps to produce serotonin and norepinephrine, which affects your emotional well-being. As you navigate the emotional terrain of pregnancy, Vitamin B6 becomes a vital ally in keeping a stable mood.

3. The Formation of Hemoglobin: Ensuring Oxygen Transport

Enter the world of hemoglobin, your blood's oxygen-carrying hero. Vitamin B6 aids in the synthesis of hemoglobin, which ensures that both you and your baby receive a proper supply of oxygen. This becomes more important as your blood volume increases throughout pregnancy, sustaining the dynamic changes in your body.

4. Morning Sickness Relief: Reducing Nausea and Vomiting

Consider Vitamin B6 to be a mild soother, helping to alleviate the waves of morning sickness that might accompany early pregnancy. This vitamin has been linked to decreased nausea and vomiting, providing a soothing touch during this transitional period.

Vitamin B6 Sources: A Culinary Palette of Nutrients

Explore the broad culinary palette that offers an abundance of Vitamin B6 as you strive to incorporate it into your diet.

1. Protein-Rich Allies: Lean Meats

Consider lean meats like chicken and turkey to be protein-rich buddies that provide your body with Vitamin B6. These meats not only contribute to your overall protein intake, but they also provide a supply of this important B-vitamin.

2. Omega-3 Harmony in Fish and Seafood

Consider fish and seafood as omega-3 fatty acid sources that complement the benefits of Vitamin B6. Salmon, tuna, and shrimp not only give vital lipids but also Vitamin B6, forming a synergistic approach to a healthy pregnancy.

3. Whole Grains: Nutrient-Dense Building Blocks

Consider whole grains, such as brown rice and oats, to be the nutrient-dense foundations that provide your body with Vitamin B6. These grains provide a diverse carbohydrate source as well as this important B-vitamin, which contributes to the overall balance of your diet.

4. Legumes: Plant-Based Superfoods

Consider legumes, such as chickpeas, lentils, and black beans, to be plant-based powerhouses high in Vitamin B6. These adaptable and nutrient-dense legumes provide a great supplement to your diet, providing protein, fiber, and important vitamins.

5. Bananas: Nature's Energy Supplements

Consider bananas to be nature's energy boosters, giving not only a quick amount of carbs but also a dosage of Vitamin B6. Bananas, as a practical and portable snack, provide a delectable way to get this crucial ingredient into your diet.

Vitamin B12: The Conductor of Cells

Change your emphasis to Vitamin B12, a vital player in the symphony of pregnancy, acting as the cellular conductor that controls numerous processes critical to the health of both you and your baby.

1. DNA Synthesis: Creating Life's Blueprint

Consider DNA synthesis to be the complex forging of life's blueprint. Vitamin B12 is essential in this process, ensuring correct DNA replication and creation. Vitamin B12 protects the genetic information that creates your baby's distinctive identity as they grow and develop rapidly.

2. Red Blood Cell Formation: Keeping Oxygen Transport Going

Consider red blood cells to be the bearers of life-sustaining oxygen, and Vitamin B12 to be the promoter of their development. This vitamin is required for the formation of red blood cells, which contributes to the oxygen delivery system that meets the needs of both your body and your kid.

3. Neurological Health: Nervous System Nourishing

In the field of neurological health, Vitamin B12 feeds the nervous system. This vitamin is essential for nerve cell health and effective communication between the brain and the rest of the body. Vitamin B12 becomes an important component in the development of your baby's neurological system.

Nature's Nutrient-Rich Offerings of Vitamin B12

Incorporate Vitamin B12 into your diet by eating a range of nutrient-rich foods.

1. Animal Products: Harmony of Meat, Fish, and Dairy

As key sources of Vitamin B12, imagine a harmonic blend of meat, fish, and dairy products. Beef, poultry, salmon, eggs, and milk all become necessary components of your diet, supplying your body with this critical B-vitamin.

2. Shellfish: Bounty of Oceanic Nutrients

Consider shellfish, such as clams, mussels, and crab, to be a marine nutrient bounty that is high in Vitamin B12. These delicacies not only add variety to your diet, but they also provide critical vitamins.

3. Fortified Foods: Nutritious Allies

Consider fortified foods like breakfast cereals and plant-based milk replacements to be enriched nutritional companions that give a source of Vitamin B12. These fortified choices represent valuable complements, particularly for vegetarian or vegan diets.

Folate: The Neural Designer

Focus on folate as you explore the realm of B-vitamins—a neural architect that plays a critical role in the development of the neural tube in early pregnancy.

1. Neural Tube Formation: Early Development Protection

Consider the early stages of pregnancy, when the neural tube forms and serves as the basis for your baby's nervous system. Folate becomes the protector of this critical process, preventing neural tube abnormalities and ensuring appropriate spinal cord closure. Adequate folate intake is especially important in the first few weeks of pregnancy, when neural growth is at its height.

2. DNA Synthesis: Life's Blueprint Continued

Consider DNA synthesis to be a continuation of life's blueprint, with folate contributing to DNA synthesis and repair. This B-vitamin is required for cell division and growth, allowing for rapid cell proliferation during pregnancy. Folate becomes a pillar in the delicate dance of life that is unfolding within you.

3. Red Blood Cell Formation: Life Oxygenation

Consider red blood cell creation to be a critical process for oxygenating life, with folate acting as a catalyst. Folate protects the

Hemoglobin production, the oxygen-carrying component of red blood cells. As the volume of your blood rises to meet the demands of pregnancy, folate becomes an essential nutrient for maintaining oxygen transport.

Folate Sources: Nature's Green Abundance

Incorporate folate into your diet by taking advantage of nature's abundant green offerings.

Verdant Nutrient Reservoirs: Leafy Greens

Consider leafy greens like spinach, kale, and collard greens to be verdant food reservoirs rich in folate. These superfoods become vital partners in achieving your folate requirements, contributing to your and your baby's general health.

Citrus Fruits: Vitamin Powerhouse

Consider citrus fruits, such as oranges, grapefruits, and lemons, to be a tangy vitamin cornucopia that provides a delightful dose of folate. These fruits not only offer flavor to your diet, but they also provide it with this important B-vitamin.

Legumes: Folate-Packed Protein Partners

Consider legumes like lentils, chickpeas, and black beans to be protein-rich folate partners that provide a double advantage for your pregnancy journey. These diverse and nutrient-dense legumes contribute significantly to your folate consumption, supporting both cellular development and protein requirements.

Fortified Foods: Improved Folate Allies

Consider fortified foods, such as cereals and grains, to be strengthened folate allies that supply an additional source of this important B-vitamin. Fortification boosts the nutritious value of these basics, making it a quick and easy option to meet your folate requirements.

A Holistic Approach to B-Vitamin Intake

When it comes to B-vitamins during pregnancy, it's critical to take a holistic approach to balancing your consumption of B6, B12, and folate. Each vitamin has a distinct yet interrelated role in the complex processes of growth, development, and well-being.

1. Nutritional Diversity: A Nutritious Tapestry

Consider dietary diversity to be a nutrient-rich tapestry that weaves together a variety of meals to supply a complete range of B-vitamins. To guarantee a well-rounded intake of B6, B12, and folate, eat a colorful and varied diet rich in fruits, vegetables, lean proteins, and whole grains.

2. Supplementation: Individual Needs Tailoring

Consider supplementing as a personalized way to meet your specific demands throughout pregnancy. Prenatal vitamins frequently contain enough quantities of B6, B12, and folate, making them an important supplement to support the particular demands of this transitional period. Consult your healthcare provider to determine the proper dosage and to confirm that supplementation is compatible with your general health.

3. Ongoing Monitoring: Promoting Well-Being

Consider regular monitoring as a caring activity to ensure your and your baby's well-being. Periodic B-vitamin levels checks can provide insight into the effectiveness of your dietary choices and supplementation, allowing for adjustments as needed.

4.   Consultation   with   Healthcare Professionals: Navigating the Path

Consider consulting with healthcare specialists to be the guiding force that guides you through the complex landscape of B-vitamins during pregnancy. Seek help from your doctor or a trained dietitian to adjust your food choices and supplementation to your unique needs, ensuring a personalized and supportive approach.

Finally, as you embark on the changing journey of pregnancy, remember the powerful impact of Vitamin B-complex—B6, B12, and folate. Consider them vital musicians in the symphony of life that is unfolding within you. You can create a holistic approach that supports both you and your growing baby through a balanced and diverse diet, thoughtful supplementation, regular monitoring, and contact with healthcare professionals. Vitamin B-complex forms a cornerstone in this harmonic orchestration of nutrients, contributing to the vivid symphony of a healthy and thriving pregnancy.

Vitamin C: Benefits and Sources

Vitamin C Advantages: Health Protector

Consider Vitamin C to be the health guardian, in the vanguard of your body's defense processes during pregnancy. This water-soluble vitamin, commonly known as ascorbic acid, provides numerous benefits that help both you and your baby.

1. Immune System Support: A Protective Barrier Against Infections

Consider Vitamin C to be a barrier that strengthens your immune system and protects you from infections and illnesses. Your body's immune defenses may fluctuate while it goes through the amazing journey of pregnancy. Vitamin C acts as an important ally, encouraging the development and function of white blood cells, improving your ability to fight infections, and assuring a strong immune response.

2. Collagen Synthesis: Maintaining Structural Integrity for You and Your Baby

Consider collagen production to be the architectural process that gives tissues, skin, and blood vessels structural integrity. Vitamin C is crucial in this process, acting as the master orchestrator of collagen formation. Vitamin C preserves the resilience and elasticity of connective tissues as your body expands and adjusts to the demands of pregnancy, contributing to the general health and vitality of both you and your baby.

3. Iron Absorption: Improving Nutrient Utilization

Consider Vitamin C to be a facilitator that improves the absorption of non-heme iron, which is found in plant-based diets and supplements. This is especially important during pregnancy, when the demand for iron increases to support blood volume expansion and the development of your baby. Vitamin C promotes efficient iron absorption, ensuring that your body uses this crucial mineral optimally and preventing iron deficiency anemia.

4. Antioxidant Defense: Free Radical Neutralization

Enter the domain of antioxidant defense, where Vitamin C serves as a scavenger, eliminating free radicals that may cause oxidative stress in your cells and your baby's. As your body changes and your baby's cells expand, Vitamin C's antioxidant qualities become important in maintaining a balanced environment, guarding against oxidative damage, and encouraging a successful pregnancy.

Vitamin C Sources: Nature's Colorful Bounty

Explore the vivid and diverse palette of foods that give a rich abundance of this crucial nutrient as you attempt to incorporate Vitamin C into your diet.

1. Citrus Fruits: Nutritious Powerhouses

Consider citrus fruits like oranges, grapefruits, lemons, and limes to be zesty vitamin C powerhouses. These fruits not only add taste to your meals, but they also provide a concentrated source of this crucial vitamin. Consider beginning your day with a glass of freshly squeezed orange juice or integrating citrus segments into salads for a tasty Vitamin C boost.

2. Berries: Antioxidant Powerhouses

Consider berries, such as strawberries, blueberries, raspberries, and blackberries, to be colorful antioxidant reservoirs that provide a tasty dose of Vitamin C. These vivid gems not only satisfy your sweet tooth, but they also contain a variety of phytonutrients and fiber, increasing the nutritional richness of your diet. Add a handful of mixed berries to yogurt, cereal, or smoothies for a delicious and nutritious treat.

3. Bell Peppers: Colorful and Crisp Vitamin C Allies

Consider bell peppers in all of their colors to be crisp and vivid Vitamin C companions that boost the nutritional profile of your meals. Bell peppers, whether red, yellow, or green, not only contribute to Vitamin C intake but also give antioxidants and important elements. Sliced bell peppers can be added to salads, stir-fries, or eaten as a crunchy snack with hummus.

4. Kiwi: Exotic Vitamin C Enchantment

Consider kiwi to be an exotic Vitamin C enchantment, providing a unique and refreshing source of this vital nutrient. Kiwi's vivid green flesh is high in Vitamin C, as well as fiber and other healthy substances. Peel and slice kiwi to enjoy as a standalone snack or to add a tropical flair to fruit salads.

5. Abundance of Tropical Vitamin C

Consider guava to be a tropical vitamin C abundance, with sweet and fragrant flesh that is high in this critical component. Guava is one of the fruits with the highest Vitamin C content, making it an important part of your pregnant diet. Fresh guava can be eaten on its own, blended into smoothies, or added to fruit salads for a tasty and nutritional boost.

6. Broccoli: A Nutritious Cruciferous Marvel

Consider broccoli to be a nutrient-dense cruciferous miracle, providing not only Vitamin C but also a variety of vitamins, minerals, and phytonutrients. This adaptable vegetable can be steamed, roasted, or stir-fried, making it a good and nourishing addition to your pregnancy meals.

7. Juicy Vitamin C Infusion from Tomatoes

Consider tomatoes to be a juicy Vitamin C infusion, whether they're eaten fresh in salads, mixed into sauces, or roasted for a burst of flavor. Tomatoes are a diverse way to get Vitamin C into your diet, as well as other healthy chemicals like lycopene, which has antioxidant characteristics.

A Wholesome Approach to Vitamin C Intake

As you traverse the various Vitamin C sources, it's critical to follow a whole-foods approach to achieve a balanced intake during pregnancy.

1. Dietary Diversity: A Nutrient Rainbow

Consider dietary diversity to be a rainbow of nutrients, with a colorful variety of fruits and vegetables providing not only Vitamin C but also a range of vitamins, minerals, and antioxidants. To improve the nutritional quality of your meals, eat a varied and balanced diet that includes a variety of citrus fruits, berries, veggies, and other Vitamin C-rich foods.

2. Cooking Methods: Nutrient Integrity Preservation

Consider cooking procedures when it comes to maintaining the nutritious integrity of vitamin C-rich meals. While some cooking methods, such as boiling, can cause the loss of water-soluble vitamins, others, such as steaming or microwaving, can assist maintain a considerable amount of Vitamin C. Experiment with various cooking procedures to find a happy medium between food safety and nutrient preservation.

3. Storage Methods: Keeping Freshness

Consider storage procedures to be freshness guardians, ensuring that vitamin C-rich foods retain their nutritious value. To maximize Vitamin C concentration, store fruits and vegetables in cool, dark places and consume them within an acceptable duration. Consider integrating fresh produce into your meals on a regular basis to reap the full nutritional benefits.

4. Supplementation: A Thoughtful Approach

Consider supplementation as a thoughtful way to supplement your food intake of Vitamin C throughout pregnancy. While acquiring nutrients from whole foods is preferable, prenatal vitamins may be a useful supplement to fill nutritional shortages. Consult your healthcare provider to establish the best dosage for your specific needs as well as general health.

5. Hydration: Vitamin C Infusion with Fluids

Consider hydration to be a fluid infusion that works in tandem with your Vitamin C consumption. Water, herbal teas, and fresh fruit juices not only meet your fluid requirements but also supply additional Vitamin C. Stay hydrated during your pregnancy as a holistic strategy that supports nutrient intake as well as overall well-being.

Healthcare Professional Consultation: Managing Your Journey

Consider consultation with healthcare specialists as the guiding force that directs your path as you embrace the benefits of Vitamin C and include its vivid sources into your pregnancy diet. Consult your healthcare professional or a qualified dietitian to adjust your Vitamin C consumption to your personal needs, taking into account aspects including individual health, food choices, and prospective supplementation.

Finally, Pregnancy Nutrition with Vitamin C

Allow Vitamin C to be your nourishing ally in the magnificent tapestry of pregnancy—a protector of health, a promoter of immunity, and a supporter of structural integrity. Recognize Vitamin C's tremendous impact on the complicated processes of growth and development as you enjoy its numerous and bright sources.

As you embark on this transforming journey, embrace the benefits of Vitamin C to ensure a well-balanced and healthy pregnancy. You may create a holistic approach that honors both you and your growing baby by being attentive to nutritional diversity, cooking methods, storage habits, hydration, and supplementation. Let Vitamin C be a harmonizing note that echoes through each stage of pregnancy nutrition, adding to the bright song of a healthy and thriving motherhood.

Vitamin D: Importance and Sun Exposure

Understanding the Importance of Vitamin D: A Health Foundation

Consider Vitamin D to be the cornerstone for good health throughout pregnancy, orchestrating a variety of processes that benefit both you and your kid. Vitamin D, also known as the "sunshine vitamin," is unique among nutrients due to its dual source—sunlight exposure and food intake.

Calcium Absorption: Bone and Teeth Strengthening

Consider calcium absorption to be the architectural process of constructing strong bones and teeth. Vitamin D functions as a facilitator, ensuring that calcium is adequately absorbed and utilized by your body. This is especially important during pregnancy, when your baby's skeletal structure is rapidly developing. Vitamin D promotes proper calcium absorption, which helps your growing baby develop a strong skeletal structure.

Immune System Regulation: A Protective Barrier Against Infections

Consider Vitamin D to be an immune system regulator, working as a barrier against infections and illnesses. This vitamin is essential for modifying immunological responses and strengthening the body's defense mechanisms. Vitamin D becomes a crucial ally as you negotiate the delicate landscape of pregnancy, where immune functions undergo dynamic transformations, supporting a resilient immune system for both you and your baby.

Cellular Differentiation and Growth: Nurturing Development

Consider cellular growth and differentiation to be the complicated processes that determine organ and tissue development. Vitamin D helps with these essential features by ensuring that cells proliferate and specialize in accordance with the life plan. Vitamin D appears as a significant role in supporting the production of critical structures throughout pregnancy, when every stage is defined by rapid growth and intricate development.

Mood Regulation: A Glimpse of Hope for Emotional Well-Being

In the field of mood modulation, Vitamin D functions as a metaphorical ray of sunlight for emotional well-being. This vitamin is linked to the manufacture of neurotransmitters such as serotonin, which is important in mood regulation. Vitamin D becomes a quiet supporter as you navigate the emotional terrain of pregnancy, potentially aiding the preservation of a balanced and pleasant mood.

Sunlight Exposure: A Natural Vitamin D Source

Consider sunshine exposure as nature's gift, offering a natural and abundant source of this critical nutrient as you investigate the importance of Vitamin D.

1. UVB Rays and Skin Synthesis: The Nutrient Offering of the Sun

Consider UVB rays as the sun's nutrient supply, kicking off an amazing process in your skin. When you expose your skin to sunlight, it produces Vitamin D3—the active form of Vitamin D. This synthesis happens in the epidermis, triggering a series of metabolic events that eventually result in the creation of Vitamin D3. This natural process demonstrates your body's balanced relationship with the sun.

2. Time of Day and Latitude: Influencing Factors in Synthesis

Consider the time of day and your geographical location as factors influencing vitamin D synthesis. Sunlight exposure at midday, when the sun is at its highest, is thought to be more beneficial for Vitamin D synthesis. Furthermore, people living at higher latitudes may have difficulty getting enough sunshine, especially during the winter months when the angle of the sun's beams is lower.

3. Skin Tone: A Sunlight Absorption Variable
Consider your skin tone to be a variable that influences solar absorption and vitamin D production. Individuals with lighter skin tones create more Vitamin D in response to sunlight exposure than individuals with darker skin tones. This discrepancy emphasizes the significance of taking into account individual variables when estimating solar exposure and Vitamin D production.

4. Exposure Duration: Balancing Benefits and Risks
Consider sunlight exposure length to be a fine balance between obtaining the benefits of Vitamin D production and avoiding the dangers associated with prolonged exposure. While some sunshine is required for Vitamin D production, excessive sun exposure can cause sunburn and raise the risk of skin cancer. Aim for a balanced approach, allowing for moderate UV exposure while taking proper measures, such as wearing sunscreen and protective clothes.

Factors Influencing Pregnancy Sunlight Exposure

Consider numerous elements that may influence your ability to receive enough Vitamin D from the sun as you negotiate the intricacies of sunlight exposure during pregnancy.

1. Seasonal Changes in Sunlight Intensity Throughout the Year

Consider seasonal fluctuations to be dynamic changes in the intensity of sunshine throughout the year. The angle of the sun's rays and the length of daylight may vary depending on the season. Obtaining proper solar exposure becomes more difficult during the winter months, especially in higher latitudes. Consider changing your schedule to maximize your exposure to sunlight during the brighter seasons, or look into alternative sources of Vitamin D during periods of low sunlight.

2. Geographical Location: Latitude and Availability of Sunlight

Consider your geographic location to be a predictor of sunshine availability, which is determined by your proximity to the equator. Individuals living in higher latitudes may have less solar exposure, especially during the winter season. Strategic planning and supplementation may be required in such circumstances to ensure appropriate Vitamin D levels throughout pregnancy.

3. Clothing Options: Modesty vs. Sun Exposure

Consider your wardrobe selections to be a factor influencing the amount of skin exposed to sunlight. While modesty and comfort are important concerns in garment choices, exposing portions of skin, such as arms and legs, might increase the efficacy of solar exposure for Vitamin D synthesis. Find a happy medium that meets your needs while allowing for adequate skin exposure.

4. Skin Protection: Considerations for Sunscreen and Sunblock

Consider skin protection to be a measure that protects against sunburn and skin damage. While sunscreen and sunblock are vital for skin health, they can also limit vitamin D synthesis. Consider using a more nuanced approach by applying sunscreen to the face and other regions prone to sunburn while allowing other portions of the body to be exposed to sunlight for brief periods before applying sunscreen.

Optimizing Sunlight Exposure During Pregnancy

Given the importance of Vitamin D and sunshine exposure, here are some suggestions for maximizing your capacity to get the advantages of sunlight while pregnant.

1. Select Optimal Sun Exposure Times: Midday Brilliance

Consider noon brilliance to be the best period for sun exposure to enhance Vitamin D production.

Aim to spend a little length of time outside during the midday sun's rays. This technique boosts the effectiveness of Vitamin D production, allowing you to reap the benefits of sunlight while reducing your risk of sunburn.

2. Expose More Skin Surface Areas: Clothing Options

Consider smart clothing choices as a technique to expose bigger areas of skin to sunlight. Choose clothing with short sleeves, skirts, or shorts to allow the arms and legs to absorb sunlight. This method allows for more skin exposure, which aids in vitamin D synthesis.

3. Think About Mindful and Moderate Sunbathing Practices

Consider sunbathing techniques to be conscious and regulated activities that support your health goals. Find a pleasant and shady outdoor area to relax and let your skin absorb sunlight. To avoid sunburn, however, be cautious of the time and intensity of your exposure. Consider the sun.

Bathing can be viewed as a comprehensive and joyful exercise that helps to your general well-being.

4. Supplementation: A Supportive Approach

Consider supplementing as a supplement to meet your Vitamin D requirements during pregnancy. While solar exposure is still the best source, supplements can be a dependable approach to ensure enough consumption, especially in situations when sunlight is scarce. Consult your healthcare provider to establish the optimal dosage for your unique needs and general health.

Health Factors to Consider: Sunlight Exposure and Skin Health

Consider health factors related to your skin and sun exposure as you investigate sunlight exposure for Vitamin D synthesis.

1. The Use of Sunscreen: Balancing Protection with Vitamin D Synthesis

Consider sunscreen to be a balancing act that protects your skin from damaging UV rays while also encouraging Vitamin D synthesis. While sunscreen is essential for avoiding sunburn and lowering the risk of skin cancer, it can also limit vitamin D production. Maintain a healthy balance by applying sunscreen to the face and other sun-sensitive areas while allowing other portions of the body to undergo brief, unprotected sun exposure.

2. Awareness and Prevention of Skin Cancer

Consider the danger of skin cancer as a factor that emphasizes the significance of sun protection. Skin cancer is increased by prolonged and unprotected sun exposure. Adopt sun-safe habits such as avoiding excessive sun exposure, using sunscreen, and wearing protective clothes to raise awareness and prevent sunburn.

3. Individual Variability: Sunlight Practice Tailoring

When adjusting solar techniques to your personal needs, keep individual heterogeneity in mind. Skin type, age, and overall health can all have an impact on how your skin reacts to sunshine. Pay attention to your body's signals and regulate your exposure to sunshine accordingly.

Healthcare Professional Consultation: Personalized Guidance

Consider consultation with healthcare specialists as a tailored guiding system as you manage the delicate balance between sunshine exposure and the need of Vitamin D during pregnancy. Consult your healthcare physician or a certified dietitian to analyze your particular needs, taking into account factors such as your health status, geographic region, and dietary habits.

Vitamin D and Sunlight for Health

Allow Vitamin D and sunlight to be your nurturing partners in the magnificent tapestry of pregnancy, building the basis for strong bones, strengthening immune resilience, fostering cellular development, and potentially contributing to pleasant mood. Recognize the significant impact of sunshine exposure on the delicate processes of growth and well-being as you bask in its advantages.

Adopt a comprehensive approach that incorporates deliberate solar exposure, smart clothing selection, health considerations, and, if necessary, supplements. Allow Vitamin D and sunlight to play harmonic notes that resound through each stage of pregnancy health, contributing to the vivid song of a healthy and thriving motherhood.

Vitamin E: Role and Food Sources

Understanding Vitamin E's Role as a Cellular Integrity Protector

Consider Vitamin E to be the defender of cellular integrity throughout pregnancy, playing a critical function in protecting your body and promoting the development of your kid. Vitamin E, as a fat-soluble antioxidant, protects against oxidative stress and is an important actor in the complicated dance of growth and well-being.

Antioxidant Defense: Free Radical Neutralization

Consider Vitamin E's antioxidant defense as a vigilant barrier, eliminating free radicals that may cause oxidative stress in your cells and those of your kid. Free radicals, which are produced by numerous metabolic processes and environmental influences, have the ability to damage cellular structures. Vitamin E acts as a defender, limiting oxidative damage and fostering a healthy environment for growth and development.

Cell Membrane Security: Maintaining Cellular Boundaries

Consider cell membranes to be delicate borders that encase the essence of life within each cell. Vitamin E helps to preserve these cell membranes and maintain their structural integrity. This is especially important during pregnancy, when cells go through dynamic changes and rapid multiplication. Vitamin E plays an important role in preserving the stability and efficiency of cells throughout your body and that of your baby by protecting cell membranes.

Immune System Support: Resilience Enhancement

Consider Vitamin E to be an immune system booster, improving its resilience and functionality. This vitamin has been linked to immune response modulation, which aids in the defense against infections and diseases. Maintaining a robust immune system becomes critical while your body navigates the challenges of pregnancy, and Vitamin E emerges as a crucial ally in this attempt.

Red Blood Cell Formation: Aiding Oxygen Transport

Consider red blood cell development to be a critical process for oxygen delivery, and Vitamin E to be a facilitator in this complex journey. Vitamin E increases the oxygen-carrying capacity of your circulation by promoting the development of red blood cells. This is especially true during pregnancy, when the demand for oxygen rises to fulfill the demands of both you and your developing baby.

Vitamin E Food Sources: A Nutrient-Rich Diet

Explore a broad and nutrient-rich palette of foods that provide ample levels of Vitamin E as you strive to incorporate it into your pregnant diet.

1. Nuts and Seeds: Powerhouses of Nutrients

Consider nuts and seeds to be nutrient-dense powerhouses that are high in Vitamin E. Almonds, sunflower seeds, hazelnuts, and pumpkin seeds are all good sources of vitamin E. Consider adding a handful of mixed nuts and seeds to your snacks or meals for a satisfying crunch and a boost of critical nutrients.

2. Culinary Elegance with Vegetable Oils

Consider vegetable oils to be culinary elegance that not only enhances the flavor of your food but also provides a good source of Vitamin E. Sunflower oil, wheat germ oil, and safflower oil are just a few of the fat-soluble vitamin-supplementing alternatives. Use these oils in cooking or as salad dressings to add flavor and nutrients to your meals.

3. Verdant Nutrient Reservoirs: Leafy Greens

Consider leafy greens like spinach, kale, and Swiss chard to be lush vitamin reservoirs bursting with Vitamin E. These superfood vegetables not only give Vitamin E but also a variety of other vitamins, minerals, and antioxidants. For a healthful and nourishing addition to your pregnant diet, use leafy greens into salads, smoothies, or sautés.

4. Fortified Foods: Better Nutritional Partners

Consider fortified goods, such as certain cereals and spreads, to be improved nutritional allies that provide additional sources of Vitamin E. These fortified alternatives can help you get more of this important nutrient, especially if you're seeking for easy methods to supplement your diet. Examine the labels of fortified items to identify them and incorporate them into your meals as part of a balanced diet.

5. Fish: Omega-3 Balance

Consider salmon and trout as sources of both Vitamin E and omega-3 fatty acids—a double harmony for your pregnancy diet. These fatty fish not only give necessary lipids, but also Vitamin E. Enjoy grilled or baked fish as a delicious and nutritious main course to diversify your diet and help the growth of your growing kid.

Fruits: Infusion of Sweet Vitamin E

Consider kiwi and mango to be a delicious Vitamin E infusion that offers a blast of taste and nutritional advantages to your diet. While fruits are not the main source of Vitamin E, they do contribute to your total intake. As a pleasant and nutritious snack to complement the broad assortment of foods on your pregnancy menu, slice up kiwi or enjoy ripe mango.

A Wholesome Approach to Vitamin E Intake

Consider taking a holistic approach to Vitamin E throughout pregnancy to guarantee a balanced intake of this key mineral.

1. Nutritional Diversity: A Nutritious Symphony

Consider dietary diversity to be a nutrient-rich symphony that weaves together numerous meals to supply a wide range of vitamins, minerals, and antioxidants, including Vitamin E. To guarantee a well-rounded intake of this fat-soluble vitamin, eat a colorful and varied diet that includes nuts, seeds, leafy greens, vegetable oils, fish, and fortified foods.

2. Cooking and Meal Planning: Maintaining Nutritional Integrity

Consider cooking and meal preparation as habits that help to keep vitamin E-rich meals nutritionally intact. While some cooking methods, such as roasting and sautéing, can preserve Vitamin E levels, others, such as deep frying, might cause losses. Experiment with different cooking processes to get the right combination of flavor, texture, and nutrient retention.

3. Storage Methods: Keeping Freshness

Consider storage procedures to be freshness guardians, ensuring that vitamin E-rich foods retain their nutritious power. Save nuts and seeds, and oils in cool, dark places to prevent oxidation and maintain the vitamin E concentration. Freshness improves the overall quality of your diet by increasing the nutritional value of these foods.

4. Supplementation: A Thoughtful Approaches

Consider supplementation as a thoughtful way to supplement your food intake of Vitamin E throughout pregnancy. While acquiring nutrients from whole foods is preferable, prenatal vitamins may be a useful supplement to fill nutritional shortages. Consult your healthcare provider to establish the optimal dosage for your unique needs and general health.

5. Healthcare Professional Consultation: Guiding the Journey

Seek the advice of healthcare specialists as you navigate the complex landscape of Vitamin E during pregnancy. Your healthcare physician or a certified dietitian can provide individualized advice based on your health state, dietary preferences, and any supplemental needs.

Finally, Pregnancy Care with Vitamin E-Rich Foods

Allow Vitamin E to be your nurturing ally in the magnificent tapestry of pregnancy—a protector of cellular integrity, an antioxidant defender, and a promoter of immune resilience. Recognize Vitamin E's enormous impact on the delicate processes of growth and development as you enjoy the numerous and nutrient-rich sources of Vitamin E.

Adopt a balanced and healthy strategy that includes a variety of Vitamin E-rich foods, as well as dietary diversity, cooking methods, storage practices, supplementation, and consultation with healthcare specialists. Let Vitamin E be a harmonizing note that echoes through each stage of pregnancy nutrition, adding to the bright song of a healthy and thriving motherhood.

Chapter 3

Essential Minerals for Expecting Mother

Iron: Vitality Building Blocks

Consider iron to be the vitality building block throughout pregnancy, an important mineral that orchestrates various fundamental tasks critical to your health and the development of your kid. Iron takes center stage in the orchestration of oxygen delivery, energy production, and overall well-being as a crucial component of hemoglobin.

1. The Importance of Hemoglobin in Oxygen Transport

Consider hemoglobin to be the oxygen-carrying hero in your bloodstream, and iron to be its essential sidekick. Hemoglobin, a protein present in red blood cells, attaches to oxygen in the lungs and distributes it to all cells in your body, maintaining a constant supply of this vital gas. Iron's role in hemoglobin is critical—without enough iron, your blood cannot carry oxygen adequately, potentially leading to iron deficiency anemia.

2. Iron's Metabolic Ballet: Energy Production

Consider iron to be a dancer in the metabolic ballet of energy creation. This mineral is essential for several cellular activities, including the synthesis of adenosine triphosphate (ATP), your cells' basic energy currency. Iron-containing enzymes aid in the conversion of nutrients into energy, giving you the energy you need to meet the demands of pregnancy.

3. Brain Development: The Impact of Iron on Neurological Health

Consider iron as a sculptor laying the groundwork for neurological health, which is especially important during pregnancy when your baby's brain is quickly developing. Iron aids in the creation of neurotransmitters, which are messengers that allow nerve cells to communicate with one another. Iron's neurological support becomes critical for your growing baby's sophisticated brain development processes.

4. Immune Function: Iron's Infection Defense

Consider iron to be a barrier that strengthens your immune system and protects you from infections and illnesses. This mineral is involved in immune cell synthesis and activity, ensuring a strong defense mechanism during pregnancy. Maintaining a strong immune system becomes increasingly important when your body experiences dynamic changes, and iron plays an important role in this protective dance.

Iron Sources: A Nutrient-Rich Symphony

Explore a symphony of nutrient-rich sources that can give this crucial element in abundance as you attempt to incorporate iron into your prenatal diet.

1. Lean Meats: Protein Powerhouses Rich in Iron

Consider lean meats like poultry, beef, and pig to be iron-rich protein powerhouses that provide a concentrated amount of this important mineral. Meat is an excellent source of iron because the heme iron found in animal-based meals is highly absorbable by the body. Consider including lean meats in your diet to maintain a sufficient quantity of iron for both you and your baby.

2. Poultry: A Versatile Iron Friend

Consider fowl, such as chicken and turkey, to be flexible iron buddies that may be used in a range of delicious ways. Poultry, whether roasted, grilled, or used in stews and stir-fries, provides not just a protein boost but also a considerable contribution to your iron needs. Investigate many ways to make fowl a delicious and nutritious addition to your pregnant menu.

3. Fish: Iron and Omega-3 Balance

Consider fish like salmon and tuna to be sources of not only iron but also omega-3 fatty acids, which are vital for your baby's brain development. These fatty fish provide a nutrient-dense choice that combines the advantages of iron with the omega-3 fatty acids contained in their meat. Grilled or baked fish is a tasty and healthful addition to any pregnant woman's diet.

4. Beans and Legumes: Iron Sources from Plants

Consider lentils, chickpeas, and black beans to be plant-powered iron sources that provide diversity and nutritional depth to your meals. While non-heme iron in plant-based foods is less easily absorbed than heme iron, pairing these foods with Vitamin C-rich choices can improve iron absorption. For a plant-based iron boost, add beans and legumes to salads, soups, or major dishes.

5. Fortified Foods: Improved Nutrition

Consider fortified foods, such as cereals and bread, to be boosted nutritional assistance with an added source of iron. Fortification includes the addition of iron to staple foods, making them easy sources of iron. Examine labels to find fortified items and incorporate them into a well-balanced diet for complete nutritional support.

6. Nuts and Seeds: Iron Allies Rich in Nutrients

Consider nuts and seeds, such as almonds, pumpkin seeds, and sunflower seeds, to be iron-rich buddies that bring a crunchy and delicious crunch to your snacks. While the iron in nuts and seeds is non-heme iron, including them in your diet helps to increase your overall iron consumption. For a delightful and nutritional boost, add a handful of mixed nuts or seeds to salads and yogurt.

7. Verdant Iron Reservoirs: Dark Leafy Greens

Consider dark leafy greens like spinach, kale, and Swiss chard to be verdant iron reservoirs that deliver a plethora of nutrients to your meal. These superfoods not only give non-heme iron but also a variety of vitamins, minerals, and antioxidants. Incorporate dark leafy greens into smoothies, salads, or sautés for a nutritious boost.

A nutritious and iron-rich supplement to your pregnant diet.

A Holistic Approach to Improving Iron Absorption

Consider a holistic strategy that involves smart dietary choices and mindful practices to improve iron absorption and guarantee that your body efficiently utilizes this crucial mineral.

1. Foods High in Vitamin C: Iron's Synergistic Partner

Consider citrus fruits, strawberries, and bell peppers to be iron's synergistic companions that improve absorption. Vitamin C promotes the conversion of non-heme iron into a more absorbable form, allowing the body to absorb it more efficiently. In your meals, combine iron-rich foods with Vitamin C sources to create a synergistic impact that promotes proper iron absorption.

2. Cooking Techniques for Maintaining Iron Integrity

Consider cooking procedures to be iron integrity guardians, protecting the nutritional content of iron-rich foods. While some cooking procedures, such as steaming and stir-frying, retain iron content, others, such as prolonged boiling, might result in iron loss. To maximize the advantages of iron-rich foods, experiment with cooking ways that find a balance between flavor, texture, and nutrient preservation.

3. Calcium Limitation and Coffee: Strategic Timing

Consider minimizing calcium-rich meals and coffee consumption as a strategy to reduce interference with iron absorption. When calcium and coffee are ingested together with iron-rich meals, they can decrease iron absorption. To encourage adequate iron absorption, plan meals strategically by avoiding calcium supplements or dairy products and refraining from drinking coffee during or immediately after meals.

4. Iron Supplementation: Seek Professional Advice

Consider iron supplementation as a consideration guided by professional guidance. While getting iron from whole foods is preferable, some people, particularly those at risk of iron deficiency, may benefit from iron supplements. Consult your healthcare professional to identify the best iron supplementation dosage and form for your specific needs and general health.

5. Ongoing Monitoring: Maintaining Iron Balance

Consider regular monitoring to maintain iron balance during your pregnancy. Periodic blood testing can help you determine your iron levels and identify any defects or abnormalities. Maintain proactive communication with your healthcare physician about your nutritional needs in order to address any issues and make informed decisions about food choices and necessary supplementation.

Iron-Rich Foods Promote Health

Allow iron to be your nurturing companion in the magnificent tapestry of pregnancy—a builder of vitality, a promoter of oxygen transport, and a protector of overall well-being. Recognize the enormous impact of iron on the intricate processes of growth and development as you enjoy the different and nutrient-rich sources of iron.

Accept a balanced and healthy approach that includes a variety of iron-rich foods, strategically blends minerals for improved absorption, and takes cooking techniques and timing into account. Allow iron to play a harmonizing note that resonates through each stage of pregnancy health, adding to the vivid song of a healthy and thriving motherhood.

Calcium: Bone Health and Fetal Development

Consider calcium to be the basis of strength throughout pregnancy, a crucial mineral that serves as the building block for bones, teeth, and a variety of physiological processes necessary for both you and your baby. The requirement for calcium increases as your body experiences dynamic changes, making it an important player in the complicated dance of bone health and fetal development.

1. The Importance of Calcium in Bone Health
Consider your bones to be the architectural structure that supports and structurally supports your body. Calcium is the foundation of this framework, and it is required to maintain bone density and strength. During pregnancy, your body's calcium requirements rise to support the formation of your baby's skeleton and to keep your own bones strong.

2. Teeth Formation: Calcium's Role in Dental Health

Consider calcium to be a sculptor who shapes the cornerstone of oral health. Calcium is essential for the production and maintenance of teeth, in addition to its involvement in bone formation. As your baby's teeth develop during pregnancy, and as your own dental health changes, having a sufficient calcium intake becomes critical in promoting strong and healthy teeth for both you and your child.

3. Muscle Function: Coordination Conductor of Calcium

Consider calcium to be the conductor in the symphony of muscle function, orchestrating the complex coordination required for muscular contractions. Calcium enables communication between neurons and muscles, providing smooth and coordinated motions from the beating of your heart to the movement of your limbs. This is especially important during pregnancy, when the demands on your muscles increase.

4. Blood Clotting: Calcium's Role in Coagulation

Consider calcium to be the coagulation maestro in the blood clotting ballet. This mineral is required for the proper operation of the blood clotting cascade, which prevents excessive bleeding in the aftermath of accidents or during childbirth. Adequate calcium levels help to maintain a delicate balance, ensuring that blood clotting occurs when needed without causing difficulties.

5. A Nutrient-Rich Symphony of Calcium Sources

Explore a symphony of nutrient-rich sources that can deliver this crucial mineral in abundance as you seek to fulfill the increased demand for calcium during pregnancy.

1. Dairy Products: Calcium-Rich Building Blocks

Consider dairy items, such as milk, yogurt, and cheese, to be calcium-rich pillars that provide a concentrated dose of this important mineral.

These dairy products not only contain a considerable quantity of calcium, but they also contain other necessary minerals such as vitamin D, which aids in calcium absorption. Include a variety of dairy products in your diet to maintain enough calcium intake for both you and your baby.

2. Verdant Calcium Reservoirs: Leafy Greens

Consider leafy greens like kale, collard greens, and broccoli to be verdant calcium reservoirs that deliver a plethora of minerals to your meal. While calcium from plant-based foods is often less absorbed than calcium from dairy, including a variety of leafy greens in your meals helps to increase your overall calcium intake. For a pleasant and healthy boost, incorporate these nutrient-dense greens into salads, soups, or sautés.

3. Fortified Foods: Better Nutritional Partners

Consider fortified foods, such as certain cereals and plant-based milk replacements, to be improved nutritional allies that supply an extra source of calcium. Fortification involves the addition of calcium to staple foods, making them practical possibilities for calcium supplementation. Examine labels to find fortified items and incorporate them into a well-balanced diet for complete nutritional support.

4. Fish: Calcium and Omega-3 Balance

Consider fish, like salmon and sardines, to be sources of not only calcium but also omega-3 fatty acids, which are vital for your baby's brain development. These fatty fish provide a nutrient-dense choice that combines the advantages of calcium with the omega-3 fatty acids contained in their meat. Grilled or baked fish is a tasty and healthful addition to any pregnant woman's diet.

5. Nuts and Seeds: Calcium-Rich Allies

Consider nuts and seeds, such as almonds, chia seeds, and sesame seeds, to be calcium buddies that bring a crunchy and delicious crunch to your snacks. While the calcium level of nuts and seeds is rather low, including them in your diet helps to increase your overall calcium consumption. For a delightful and nutritional boost, add a handful of mixed nuts or seeds to salads and yogurt.

A Developmental Ballet on Calcium and Fetal Development

Recognize the critical role that calcium plays in building the skeletal foundation and supporting numerous physiological processes as you nurture your baby's growth and development.

1. Skeletal Formation: Calcium's Bone Blueprint

Consider calcium to be the architect who is creating the plan for your baby's skeletal structure. Your baby's bones develop rapidly during pregnancy, with the skeleton serving as the framework for future growth. A sufficient calcium intake ensures that this developmental process proceeds properly, supplying the necessary building blocks for strong and durable bones.

2. Calcium's Cardiovascular Role in Intrauterine Blood Circulation

Consider calcium to be the conductor of intrauterine blood circulation, vital to the development of your baby's cardiovascular system. Calcium helps to create the heart and blood arteries, which ensures appropriate functioning and the construction of an effective circulatory system. This cardiovascular support becomes the bedrock for your baby's entire health.

3. Neurological Development: The Effect of Calcium on the Nervous System

Consider calcium to be the directing force in fetal development's neuronal ballet. This mineral regulates the creation and function of the neurological system, ensuring normal brain and nerve development. The availability of calcium becomes important in creating the basis for cognitive and motor functions as your baby's brain connections take development.

4. Muscle Function: Coordination of Calcium in Tiny Limbs

Consider calcium to be the muscular function coordinator in your baby's tiny limbs, allowing for coordinated motions and muscle contractions. Calcium enhances nerve-muscle communication as the musculoskeletal system develops, setting the framework for the precise motions your baby will exhibit both in gestation and after birth.

A Holistic Approach to Calcium Absorption

Consider using a comprehensive strategy that considers dietary choices, lifestyle behaviors, and potential factors that may influence calcium absorption to ensure that your body absorbs and utilizes the calcium you ingest properly.

1. Vitamin D Synergy: Collaboration for Absorption

Consider Vitamin D to be a synergistic partner who improves calcium absorption. Vitamin D is essential for calcium metabolism because it promotes calcium absorption from the intestines into the circulation. To maximize the synergistic link between Vitamin D and calcium, get enough sunlight, eat vitamin D-rich foods, or consider supplementing.

2. Adequate Magnesium Intake: A Fine Balance

Consider magnesium intake to be a balancing act that promotes proper calcium absorption. Magnesium collaborates with calcium to regulate calcium transit and usage inside the body. To maintain a harmonious balance that leads to good calcium absorption, incorporate magnesium-rich foods in your diet, such as nuts, seeds, and whole grains.

3. Limitation Caffeine and Sodium: Maintaining Balance

Consider decreasing your intake of caffeine and sodium as a strategy that supports calcium absorption equilibrium. Caffeine and sodium intake in excess can interfere with calcium absorption and lead to calcium loss through urine. Caffeinated beverages and processed meals should be consumed in moderation to ensure a balanced approach to calcium absorption.

4. Regular Exercise: Bone Health Maintenance

Consider regular exercise to be a bone health protector, promoting the efficient usage of calcium inside the skeletal system. Weight-bearing workouts like walking, running, and strength training help to increase bone density and strength. Include regular physical activity in your daily routine to improve calcium utilization and overall bone health during pregnancy.

Finally, Calcium Promotes Strength and Development

Let calcium be your nurturing friend in the magnificent tapestry of pregnancy—a foundation of strength, a promoter of bone health, and an essential contributor to fetal development. Recognize the significant impact of calcium on the complicated processes of growth and well-being as you enjoy the different and nutrient-rich sources of calcium.

Adopt a balanced and healthy strategy that includes a variety of calcium-rich meals, factors impacting absorption, and lifestyle activities that promote bone health. Allow calcium to play a harmonizing note that echoes through each stage of pregnancy, contributing to the bright song of a healthy and thriving motherhood.

Zinc: Functions and Dietary Sources

Zinc is a cellular conductor, conducting a symphony of functions critical to your health and the growth of your kid throughout pregnancy. As a trace mineral, zinc participates in a wide range of physiological processes that go far beyond its humble presence, contributing to the subtle dance of growth, immunity, and overall health.

1. Zinc's Architectural Role in Cellular Growth and Division

Consider zinc to be the architect in charge of cellular growth and division, which is essential during pregnancy. This mineral is essential for the synthesis of DNA, RNA, and proteins, as well as the development and reproduction of cells. As your infant grows, zinc becomes an important role in the formation of the complicated structures that serve as the foundation for growth.

2. Immune Function: Zinc's Infection Defense

Consider zinc to be a shield that strengthens your immune system and protects both you and your baby from infections. This mineral promotes immune cell activity, aids in antibody synthesis, and aids in the maintenance of the skin and mucous membranes—barriers that serve as the first line of defense against infections. Maintaining a strong immune system becomes critical while your body navigates the challenges of pregnancy, and zinc is an important ally in this attempt.

3. Zinc's Catalyst Role in Enzyme Activity

Consider zinc to be a catalyst that drives enzymatic activity, which is a critical component of many metabolic reactions in your body. Many enzymes, which aid in vital functions like digestion and metabolism, rely on zinc as a cofactor. Zinc contributes to the effectiveness of physiological activities by boosting enzymatic activity, ensuring that your body runs smoothly during the complex trip of pregnancy.

4. Wound Healing: The Repairing Touch of Zinc

Consider zinc as a restorative touch in the complex process of wound healing. This mineral aids in tissue repair and regeneration by assisting in the healing of injured cells and the production of new tissue. As your body develops and adapts during pregnancy, zinc's capacity to help wound healing becomes increasingly important.

A Nutrient-Rich Palette of Zinc Sources

Explore a broad and nutrient-rich palette of foods that serve as good sources of zinc during pregnancy to ensure that you satisfy the increased need for this critical mineral.

1. Meat and Seafood: Protein Powerhouses High in Zinc

Consider cattle, pork, lamb, and shellfish to be zinc-rich protein powerhouses that provide a concentrated amount of this critical mineral. Animal-based zinc sources, known as heme sources, have a high bioavailability, making them good candidates for increasing your zinc consumption. Include a variety of meats and seafood in your diet to provide a steady supply of zinc for you and your baby.

2. Nuts and Seeds: Zinc-Dense Allies

Consider nuts and seeds, such as pumpkin seeds, cashews, and almonds, to be zinc allies that bring a crunchy and delicious crunch to your snacks. While the zinc level of plant-based foods is less absorbable than that of animal sources, including a variety of nuts and seeds in your diet helps to increase your overall zinc intake. For a delightful and nutritional boost, add a handful of mixed nuts or seeds to salads and yogurt.

3. Legumes: Zinc Sources from Plants

Consider legumes like lentils, chickpeas, and beans to be plant-powered zinc sources that provide diversity and nutritional richness to your diet. While non-heme zinc in plant-based meals may be less easily absorbed, supplementing these foods with sources of Vitamin C can improve zinc absorption. For a plant-based zinc boost, add legumes to soups, stews, or salads.

4. Dairy Products: Zinc from Calcium-Rich Alternatives

Consider dairy items such as milk, yogurt, and cheese to be zinc sources that also include a plethora of critical minerals such as calcium. While dairy products are not the primary source of zinc, they do contribute to your daily consumption. Enjoy a variety of dairy products as part of a balanced diet, keeping in mind their function in not only providing zinc but also meeting other nutritional demands during pregnancy.

5. Whole Grains: Zinc-Rich Allies

Consider whole grains like quinoa, oats, and whole wheat to be zinc-rich companions that make a healthy complement to your diet. While whole grains include non-heme zinc, including them in your diet helps to increase your overall zinc consumption. To increase the nutritious diversity of your pregnancy diet, use whole grains as a foundation for meals, such as salads, stir-fries, or as a side dish.

6. Eggs: Zinc in a Nutritious Package

Consider eggs to be a nutrient-dense package that contains zinc as well as a variety of other necessary elements. Eggs are an excellent source of zinc because they include not only this essential mineral but also proteins, vitamins, and healthy fats. Include eggs in your diet in a variety of ways, including omelets, scrambles, and as a protein-rich addition to salads.

A Strategic Approach to Zinc Absorption

Consider a strategic strategy that integrates dietary choices and factors influencing zinc absorption to improve zinc absorption and guarantee that your body effectively utilizes this critical mineral.

1. By combining with vitamin C, you can improve absorption

Consider combining zinc-rich foods with vitamin C-rich alternatives to improve absorption. Vitamin C aids in the absorption of non-heme zinc, which is abundant in plant foods. Combine zinc-rich foods with vitamin C-rich fruits and vegetables such as citrus fruits, strawberries, bell peppers, or broccoli to make colorful and tasty meals.

2. Cooking Methods for Maintaining Zinc Integrity

Consider cooking processes to be zinc integrity guardians, protecting the nutritional content of zinc-rich foods. While some cooking processes, such as roasting and sautéing, preserve zinc levels, others, such as boiling, may result in losses. To maximize the advantages of zinc-rich foods, experiment with cooking ways that create a balance between flavor, texture, and nutrient preservation.

3. A Mindful Approach to Limiting Phytates

Consider decreasing your intake of phytates as a thoughtful strategy that may improve zinc absorption. Phytates, which exist naturally in several plant-based meals, can bind to zinc and impede its absorption. While phytates provide health benefits, try diversifying your diet with zinc-rich foods and keeping overall nutritional balance in mind.

4. Protein Presence: Aiding Absorption

Consider protein in your meals to be a helpful component in zinc absorption. Protein aids zinc absorption in the intestines, increasing the overall efficiency of the process. Make careful to combine zinc-rich foods with protein sources in your meals to generate a synergistic impact that supports healthy zinc absorption.

A Nutritional Ballet of Zinc and Pregnancy

Recognize the critical function zinc plays in supporting both your health and the development of your baby as you travel through the delicate path of pregnancy.

1. Fetal Growth and Development: Zinc's Cellular Blueprint

Consider zinc to be the architect who creates the blueprint for your baby's cellular growth and development. Zinc aids in the production of DNA and proteins, creating the groundwork for cell creation and replication. Adequate zinc intake is critical for the complicated processes that shape your baby's cells and tissues.

2. Immune Support: Zinc's Protector Role

Consider zinc to be a protector who strengthens your baby's immune system, which is an important part of general health. Zinc's significance in immune function extends to the growing newborn, where it aids in the creation of immune cells and the establishment of a durable defense mechanism. As your baby's immune system develops, zinc becomes increasingly important in this protective dance.

3. Neurological Development: The Effect of Zinc on the Nervous System

Consider zinc to be a player in the cerebral ballet of fetal development. This mineral aids in the development and function of the nervous system, helping to create the brain and nerves. As your baby's brain pathways develop, zinc availability becomes important in laying the groundwork for cognitive and motor functions.

4. Wound Healing: Zinc's Role in Tissue Repair

Consider zinc as a component of your baby's developing body's complicated wound healing process. Zinc's role in tissue repair becomes increasingly important as cells grow and differentiate. This mending touch extends to your baby's developing tissues and organs, enabling a smooth developmental path.

Zinc-Rich Foods Promote Health

Allow zinc to be your nurturing ally in the magnificent tapestry of pregnancy—a cellular conductor, a development architect, and a protector of overall well-being. Recognize the significant impact of zinc on the delicate processes of fetal development and your own health as you enjoy the different and nutrient-rich sources of zinc.

Accept a balanced and healthy strategy that includes a variety of zinc-rich meals, strategically blends nutrients for improved absorption, and takes into account aspects impacting total dietary balance. Allow zinc to play a harmonizing note that resonates through each stage of pregnancy nutrition, contributing to the vivid song of a healthy and successful motherhood.

Magnesium: Importance During Pregnancy

Magnesium to be a vital symphony conductor, directing a plethora of functions critical to your health and the growth of your kid during pregnancy. Magnesium emerges as a silent hero as a mineral involved in over 300 enzymatic activities within your body, contributing to the complicated dance of growth, energy production, and overall well-being.

1. Magnesium's Metabolic Spark: Energy Production

Consider magnesium to be the metabolic spark that ignites energy production within your cells. This mineral is essential in the conversion of foods, such as carbs and fats, into usable energy, ensuring that you have the vitality required to support the dynamic changes that occur during pregnancy. Magnesium becomes more important as your body adjusts to the higher energy demands of caring for a growing baby.

2. Muscle Function: Magnesium's Master of Coordination

Consider magnesium to be the maestro of coordination in the symphony of muscular activity, enabling muscle contraction and relaxation. Magnesium enables the seamless synchronization of muscle function, from the rhythmic pounding of your heart to the delicate movements of your limbs. As your body changes and your baby grows throughout pregnancy, the importance of magnesium in sustaining muscular function becomes critical.

3. Bone Health: Magnesium's Role in Skeletal Integrity

Consider magnesium to be a contributor to skeletal integrity, acting in tandem with other minerals such as calcium. While calcium is generally the focus of bone health discussions, magnesium also plays an important role in bone production and density. Magnesium becomes an unsung hero as your baby's skeleton develops, adding to the strength and structure of both your bones and those of your growing kid.

4. Neurological System Regulation: Magnesium's Calming Effect

Consider magnesium to be a calming effect on the nervous system, aiding in stress regulation and relaxation. This mineral influences neurotransmitters, which are messengers that send impulses between nerve cells. Magnesium helps a balanced nerve system as you manage the emotional and physical changes of pregnancy, contributing to a sense of peace and well-being.

5. Magnesium's Vascular Harmony: Blood Pressure Regulation

Consider magnesium to be a defender of vascular harmony, helping to regulate blood pressure. This mineral aids in vasodilation, or the widening of blood vessels, which aids in the maintenance of healthy blood pressure levels. When blood volume and circulation fluctuate during pregnancy, magnesium's influence on vascular function becomes critical for general cardiovascular well-being.

A Nutrient-Rich Palette of Magnesium Sources

Explore a broad and nutrient-rich palette of foods that serve as good sources of magnesium to ensure that you fulfill the increased need for this crucial mineral during pregnancy.

Verdant Magnesium Reservoirs: Leafy Greens

Consider leafy greens like spinach, kale, and Swiss chard to be verdant magnesium reservoirs that deliver a plethora of nutrients to your meal. These superfoods not only give magnesium but also a variety of vitamins, minerals, and antioxidants. Dark leafy greens can be added to salads, smoothies, or cooked dishes for a delicious and nutritional boost.

Nuts and Seeds: Magnesium Allies Rich in Nutrients

Consider nuts and seeds, such as almonds, pumpkin seeds, and sunflower seeds, to be magnesium allies that bring a crunchy and delicious crunch to your snacks. These magnesium-rich choices also contain beneficial fats and other nutrients. For a delightful and nutritious boost, add a handful of mixed nuts or seeds to salads, yogurt, or oatmeal.

Whole Grains: Magnesium in Nutritious Forms

Consider healthy grains like quinoa, brown rice, and oats to be magnesium-rich components of nutritious meals. Whole grains not only provide magnesium but also fiber, vitamins, and minerals to your diet. For a nutrient-rich and fulfilling experience, use whole grains as a base for foods like salads, stir-fries, or grain bowls.

Legumes: Magnesium Sources from Plants

Consider legumes, such as lentils, chickpeas, and black beans, to be plant-powered magnesium sources that add diversity and nutritional richness to your diet. These magnesium-rich legumes also provide protein and fiber, which help to maintain overall dietary balance. For a plant-based magnesium boost, make healthy soups, stews, or salads with legumes.

Fish: Magnesium and Omega-3 Balance

Consider fish like salmon and mackerel as sources of not only magnesium but also the necessary omega-3 fatty acids required for your baby's brain development. These fatty fish provide a nutrient-dense choice that combines magnesium's benefits with the omega-3s contained in their meat. Grilled or baked fish is a tasty and healthful addition to any pregnant woman's diet.

A Nutritional Ballet of Magnesium and Pregnancy

Recognize the critical function that magnesium plays in supporting both your health and the development of your baby as you travel through the delicate path of pregnancy.

1. Fetal Growth and Development: Magnesium's Role in Cellular Function

Consider magnesium as a player in the cellular orchestra that shapes your baby's growth and development. This mineral aids in the development and replication of cells by participating in DNA and RNA synthesis. Adequate magnesium intake is critical in ensuring the complicated processes that establish the groundwork for your baby's cellular architecture.

2. Magnesium's Metabolic Harmony: Energy Production for Both

Consider magnesium to be a metabolic process stabilizer, ensuring the creation of energy for both you and your growing kid. Magnesium aids in the metabolic events that occur when your body metabolizes nutrients to generate energy. During pregnancy, its presence becomes increasingly important, providing the metabolic spark required to meet the increased energy demands of caring for a developing baby.

3. Magnesium's Influence on Muscle and Nervous System Development

Consider magnesium as a factor in your baby's muscular and nervous system development. This mineral helps to coordinate muscle activity and controls neurotransmitters, resulting in a well-balanced and well-functioning musculoskeletal and neural system. As your baby's body develops, magnesium's participation in these developmental features becomes increasingly important.

4. Skeletal Integrity: Magnesium's Bone Support

Consider magnesium to be a skeletal integrity supporter, aiding in the development of your baby's bones. While calcium is frequently discussed in relation to bone health, magnesium also contributes to bone growth and density, ensuring that your baby's skeleton grows strong and durable. The combination of magnesium and other minerals becomes critical for the overall health of growing bones.

5. Magnesium's Cardiovascular Influence on Blood Pressure

Consider magnesium to be a cardiovascular health guardian, helping to regulate blood pressure in both you and your baby. During pregnancy, the role of this mineral on vasodilation and blood vessel function becomes critical, supporting optimal blood pressure levels. Magnesium is an important ally in preserving cardiovascular harmony as your body's blood volume and circulation vary.

How to Improve Magnesium Absorption: A Strategic Plan

Consider a strategic strategy that takes into consideration dietary choices, lifestyle behaviors, and factors impacting magnesium absorption to ensure that your body absorbs and utilizes the magnesium you consume properly.

1. A Nutrient-Rich Ensemble: A Balanced Diet

Consider a balanced diet to be a nutrient-dense ensemble that promotes total magnesium absorption. A varied array of nutrients is ensured by consuming a variety of magnesium-rich meals, generating a synergistic impact that improves absorption. To enhance magnesium absorption, eat a well-balanced diet rich in vegetables, fruits, whole grains, nuts, seeds, and lean meats.

2. Vitamin D Synergy: Collaboration for Absorption

Consider Vitamin D to be a synergistic partner that boosts magnesium absorption. Vitamin D aids in magnesium metabolism by boosting absorption from the intestines into the circulation. To maximize the synergistic interaction between Vitamin D and magnesium, get appropriate sunlight exposure, consume Vitamin D-rich foods, or consider supplementing.

3. A Careful Approach to Calcium Supplementation

Consider reducing calcium dosage as a deliberate strategy that may improve magnesium absorption. While both elements are necessary for bone health, too much calcium may interfere with magnesium absorption. Consult your healthcare professional to discover the best balance of calcium and magnesium supplementation for your specific needs and health status.

4. Controlling Caffeine and Alcohol Absorption

Consider coffee and alcohol use as a beneficial habit for magnesium absorption. Caffeine and alcohol use can increase magnesium excretion through the urine. To maintain a healthy magnesium level throughout pregnancy, consume caffeinated beverages and alcoholic beverages with caution.

5. Adequate Hydration: Beneficial for Nutrient Transport

Consider proper hydration as a nutrient transport facilitator, including magnesium. Staying hydrated helps nutrients, including magnesium, travel through the circulation to cells and tissues.

Maintain optimal hydration levels by drinking plenty of water throughout the day, which will aid in the efficient delivery of magnesium to cells.

Magnesium-Rich Foods Promote Vitality

Allow magnesium to be your nurturing ally in the magnificent tapestry of pregnancy—a vital symphony conductor, a metabolic spark, and a protector of overall well-being. Recognize magnesium's enormous impact on the delicate processes of growth and development as you enjoy the numerous and nutrient-rich sources of magnesium.

Accept a balanced and healthy approach that includes a variety of magnesium-rich meals, strategically blends minerals for improved absorption, and takes into account aspects impacting total dietary balance. Allow magnesium to play a harmonizing note that resonates through each stage of pregnancy nutrition, contributing to the vivid song of a healthy and successful motherhood.

Chapter 4

Special Considerations and Supplements

Understanding Omega-3 Fatty Acids

Omega-3 fatty acids are considered to be nature's food, necessary for the delicate dance of growth, development, and overall health during pregnancy. Omega-3 fatty acids, which are classified into three types—ALA (alpha-linolenic acid), EPA (eicosapentaenoic acid), and DHA (docosahexaenoic acid)—play critical roles in a variety of physiological processes, making them invaluable companions in the adventure of raising a new life.

1. DHA's Cognitive Symphony for Brain Development

Consider DHA to be the conductor of a cognitive symphony, orchestrating the growth of your baby's brain during pregnancy. This omega-3 fatty acid is a structural component of brain tissue that influences neuronal networks and aids cognitive function. Adequate DHA intake is especially important during the last trimester, when the baby's brain grows rapidly, establishing the groundwork for future cognitive abilities.

2. Visual Acuity: Ocular Elegance of DHA

Consider DHA to be the maestro who enhances the ocular elegance of your baby's vision. This omega-3 fatty acid is an important component of the retina, promoting eye development and visual acuity. Including DHA in your diet throughout pregnancy aids with the development of the delicate structures that determine your baby's capacity to see and perceive the environment.

3. EPA's Cardiovascular Harmony: Heart Health

Consider EPA to be the cardiovascular harmony maintainer, supporting both your and your baby's heart health during pregnancy. This omega-3 fatty acid helps to reduce inflammation, regulate blood clotting, and promote overall cardiovascular health. EPA's effect becomes a key contributor to a healthy heart while your body undergoes changes in blood volume and circulation throughout pregnancy.

4. The ALA's Balancing Act on Inflammatory Response

Consider ALA to be the balancing act in the symphony of inflammatory response, helping to manage inflammation management. While ALA is a precursor to EPA and DHA, it also has anti-inflammatory benefits on its own. Maintaining equilibrium in inflammatory processes becomes critical during pregnancy, and ALA's presence adds a layer of support.

A Bounty of Nutrient-Rich Omega-3 Fatty Acid Sources

To ensure that you reap the benefits of omega-3 fatty acids throughout pregnancy, look into a variety of nutrient-rich options that are high in these vital fats.

1. Oceanic Omega-3 Rich Fatty Fish

Consider fatty fish like salmon, mackerel, sardines, and trout to be marine omega-3 treasures that provide a concentrated amount of EPA and DHA. These fatty fish are a nutrient-dense option, combining omega-3 fatty acid advantages with high-quality proteins and other critical components. Grilled or baked fish is a tasty and healthful addition to any pregnant woman's diet.

2. Chia Seeds: ALA Nutrient Allies

Consider chia seeds to be ALA buddies that provide a plant-based source of omega-3 fatty acids. These small seeds pack a powerful nutritional punch, containing a high concentration of ALA as well as fiber and other vital minerals. Chia seeds can be added to yogurt, smoothies, or oatmeal for a delightful and omega-3-rich boost to your meals.

3. Walnuts: ALA Crunchy Powerhouses

Consider walnuts to be crunchy ALA powerhouses that provide texture and nutritional richness to your snacks. Walnuts contain a significant quantity of ALA, making them an easy and delicious source of omega-3 fatty acids. Enjoy a handful of walnuts as a snack or sprinkle them on salads, cereals, or desserts for a tasty and omega-3-rich addition.

4. Flaxseeds: Super Seeds High in ALA

Consider flaxseeds to be ALA-rich super seeds that help you get enough omega-3 fatty acids. These flexible seeds are high in ALA and can be easily incorporated into a variety of meals. Ground flaxseeds can be added to smoothies, baked products, or sprinkled on salads and yogurt to improve your omega-3 levels.

5. Plant-Powered DHA Algal Oil Supplements
Consider algal oil supplements to be plant-powered DHA sources produced from algae. Algal oil is a vegan-friendly alternative to fish oil, and it provides a direct source of DHA. Consider include algal oil supplements in your regimen to guarantee a regular and adequate dose of this important omega-3 fatty acid during pregnancy.

Pregnancy and Omega-3 Fatty Acids: A Nutritional Symphony

Recognize the critical function that omega-3 fatty acids play in supporting both your health and the optimal development of your baby as you travel through the delicate journey of pregnancy.

1. Cognitive Development: DHA's Brilliance Blueprint

Consider DHA to be the architect who creates the blueprint for your baby's cognitive growth.

This omega-3 fatty acid alters brain structure and function, promoting neuronal pathway creation and laying the groundwork for future cognitive ability. Adequate DHA consumption plays an important role in nourishing the brilliance that will emerge as your baby's brain develops.

2. Visual Acuity: DHA's Vision Artistry

Consider DHA to be the artist who creates the creativity of your baby's vision. This omega-3 fatty acid promotes eye growth and improves visual acuity, guaranteeing that your baby's vision is a work of art. The presence of DHA becomes critical for the delicate process of visual development as the retina takes shape and the eyes begin to perceive light.

3. EPA's Melody of Harmony for Cardiovascular Support

Consider EPA to be the harmonious melody that promotes cardiovascular health in both you and your kid. This omega-3 fatty acid helps to reduce inflammation, regulate blood clotting, and promote general cardiovascular health. As your baby's heart develops and your own cardiovascular system changes during pregnancy, EPA's influence becomes a soothing song.

4. ALA's Symphony of Equilibrium: Anti-Inflammatory Balance

Consider ALA to be a symphony conductor, orchestrating the balance of inflammatory response throughout pregnancy. While ALA is a precursor to EPA and DHA, it also has anti-inflammatory qualities on its own, helping to maintain the delicate balance essential for a balanced inflammatory response. Striking this balance becomes especially important during pregnancy, since it promotes overall well-being.

A Strategic Approach to Improving Omega-3 Fatty Acid Absorption

Consider a strategic strategy that integrates dietary choices, supplements, and factors influencing absorption to improve omega-3 fatty acid absorption and use.

1.   Balanced   Diet: Nutrient-Dense Composition

Consider a balanced diet to be a nutrient-dense composition that promotes overall omega-3 fatty acid absorption. Consuming a varied array of omega-3-rich foods assures a diverse array of nutrients, resulting in a synergistic impact that improves absorption. To maximize absorption, aim for a balanced and healthful diet that contains a variety of fatty fish, seeds, nuts, and other omega-3 sources.

2. Regular Fish Consumption: A Marine Nutrient Routine

Consider integrating frequent fish consumption in your diet to ensure a steady intake of marine nutrients such as EPA and DHA. Fatty fish provide a direct source of omega-3 fatty acids in a natural and accessible form that aids absorption. To guarantee a continuous supply, aim for at least two servings of fatty fish every week.

3. Supplementation: A Reliable Source of Omega-3

Consider omega-3 supplementation to be a dependable source for filling any gaps and ensuring constant consumption of these vital fatty acids. Fish oil or algal oil capsules, for example, are a handy and controlled approach to receive EPA and DHA. Consult your healthcare practitioner to identify the best supplement regimen for your specific needs and health status.

4. Cooking Techniques: Nutrient Integrity Preservation

Consider cooking processes to be nutrient integrity defenders, protecting foods' omega-3 content. While some cooking methods, such as grilling and baking, preserve omega-3 fatty acids, others, such as deep frying, may deplete them. To enhance the nutritional value of omega-3-rich foods, experiment with cooking procedures that preserve their nutritious worth.

5. Storage Practices: Oxidation Protection

Consider storage procedures to be oxidation barriers that safeguard the integrity of omega-3 fatty acids in foods and supplements. Light, heat, and air exposure can all contribute to the oxidation of these delicate fats. Store omega-3-rich meals in cold, dark settings, and follow supplement storage directions to keep them fresh and effective.

Finally, Omega-3-Rich Foods Can Help You Live Longer

Allow omega-3 fatty acids to be your loving companions in the magnificent tapestry of pregnancy—nature's nourishment, architects of brilliance, and melodies of harmony. Recognize the deep impact of these important fats on the intricate processes of growth and development as you appreciate the different and nutrient-rich sources of these vital fats.

Adopt a balanced and healthy strategy that integrates a variety of omega-3-rich foods, evaluates the benefits of supplementation, and takes into account factors impacting total dietary balance. Allow omega-3 fatty acids to play a harmonizing note that resonates through each stage of pregnancy nutrition, contributing to the bright song of a healthy and flourishing motherhood.

Prenatal Multivitamins: Nutrition for Two

Consider prenatal multivitamins to be customized nutrition for both you and your growing baby, giving a full array of critical vitamins and minerals necessary for a successful pregnancy. As your body changes to support new life, the demand for specific nutrients rises, and prenatal multivitamins serve an important role in filling potential gaps to support overall well-being.

1. Folic Acid: The Building Block of Neural Tube Development

Consider folic acid to be the foundation for neural tube development, which is critical throughout the early stages of pregnancy. This B-vitamin is important in preventing neural tube abnormalities in the spine and brain of a developing baby. A high-quality prenatal multivitamin has an adequate dose of folic acid, which provides vital support throughout the critical period of neural tube formation.

2. Iron: Vital Oxygenation for Both

Consider iron to be the oxygenating vigor that both you and your baby require. Iron is necessary for preventing iron deficiency anemia, which can cause fatigue and reduce the blood's oxygen-carrying ability. Maintaining adequate iron levels becomes critical during pregnancy, when blood volume increases to support the growing baby. A prenatal multivitamin containing iron guarantees that both you and your baby get this essential nutrient.

3. Calcium for Skeletal Health

Consider calcium to be the defender of your and your baby's skeletal health. This mineral is essential for the growth of the baby's bones and teeth. Furthermore, calcium promotes your own bone health during pregnancy. A well-rounded prenatal multivitamin contains a suitable amount of calcium, which contributes to your and your growing baby's overall skeletal well-being.

4. Vitamin D: Collaboration for Calcium Absorption

Consider vitamin D to be the partner who aids calcium absorption—a dynamic combo for bone health. While calcium is necessary, vitamin D improves absorption, ensuring that both you and your baby benefit. A prenatal multivitamin containing vitamin D supplements calcium intake, promoting proper usage of this essential mineral.

5. Omega-3 Fatty Acids: Brain and Vision Support

Consider omega-3 fatty acids to be brain and visual development nourishment. DHA, a form of omega-3 fatty acid, is essential for the brain and eyes of a developing newborn. DHA may be included in a high-quality prenatal multivitamin, providing an additional source of this critical fatty acid to enhance cognitive and visual development.

6. Iodine and Thyroid Function and Cognitive Development

Consider iodine to be a thyroid function and cognitive development regulator. Adequate iodine consumption is required for the production of thyroid hormones, which play a role in general metabolism. Furthermore, iodine is necessary for the cognitive function of a developing baby. Iodine is included in a comprehensive prenatal multivitamin to promote both your thyroid health and your baby's cognitive development.

7. Vitamin B12: Formation of Red Blood Cells and Nervous System Support

Consider vitamin B12 to be an aid to red blood cell development and nervous system wellness. This vitamin is necessary for the synthesis of red blood cells, the prevention of anemia, and the proper functioning of the brain system. A well-formulated prenatal multivitamin offers an adequate supply of vitamin B12 for the health of both you and your baby.

A Strategic Approach to Choosing the Best Prenatal Multivitamin

Consider taking a strategic approach that takes individual circumstances, dietary habits, and health issues into account when selecting the correct prenatal multivitamin tailored to your personal needs.

1. Consultation with a Healthcare Provider: Individualized Advice

Consider a meeting with your healthcare professional as a compass pointing you in the right direction. Discuss your individual health status, dietary habits, and special needs with your healthcare practitioner before selecting a prenatal multivitamin. They can make personalized suggestions based on pre-existing conditions, dietary limitations, and probable vitamin deficits.

2. Assessing Individual Nutrient Requirements

Consider your particular nutrient requirements as the starting point for determining your specific requirements. Age, food choices, and current nutrient levels all play a part in determining which vitamins and minerals may require supplementation. A prenatal multivitamin tailored to your specific needs provides focused assistance for both you and your baby.

3. Nutritional Dosage: Finding the Right Balance

Consider nutrient doses to be the delicate balance in selecting the best prenatal multivitamin. While it is critical to meet increased dietary requirements during pregnancy, excessive dosages may pose dangers. Choose a prenatal multivitamin that contains enough, but not excessive, amounts of vital nutrients to ensure that you achieve the correct balance between safety and effectiveness.

4. Bioavailability: Nutrient Absorption Optimization

Consider bioavailability to be the enhancement of nutrient absorption, which improves the effectiveness of your chosen prenatal multivitamin. Some vitamins and minerals are better absorbed by the body than others. Select a prenatal multivitamin that contains bioavailable forms of nutrients to promote maximum absorption and utilization for both you and your baby.

5. Comprehensive Formulation: All Bases Covered

Consider a comprehensive formulation to be the canopy that covers all bases, guaranteeing that your chosen prenatal multivitamin addresses a wide range of nutrient requirements. Look for a multivitamin that has a wide range of vitamins and minerals, covering the necessities for both you and your kid's well-being. A well-rounded composition helps to support the holistic approach that is required during pregnancy.

6. Quality and Purity: Assurance of Safety

Consider quality and purity to be the defenders of the safety of your prenatal multivitamin pick. Choose a renowned brand that complies to severe quality control methods, such as third-party purity and potency testing. Choosing a high-quality prenatal multivitamin reduces the chance of contamination while also ensuring that you are receiving a safe and effective supplement.

7. Considering Dietary Habits: Filling Gaps

Consider your food choices to be the canvas on which your prenatal multivitamin supplements will be able to fill any holes. If your diet is lacking in specific nutrients, a prenatal multivitamin can address those gaps, ensuring that you and your baby get a full range of critical vitamins and minerals. Align your supplement selection with your eating habits for a balanced and supportive approach.

Finally, the Right Prenatal Multivitamin Can Help You Have a Healthy Pregnancy

Allow the correct prenatal multivitamin to be your personalized ally in the magnificent tapestry of pregnancy, supplying important nutrients, promoting general well-being, and contributing to the optimal growth of your growing baby. Consider the strategic approach of selecting a prenatal multivitamin that matches with your particular needs as you embark on this transforming journey, assuring a harmonious and effective supplement for a healthy and successful pregnancy.

Herbal Supplements: Caution and Consideration

Consider herbal supplements to be threads sewn into the historical tapestry of traditional medicine, providing a varied range of plants with alleged therapeutic characteristics. Herbs have been used for healing and well-being by societies all over the world throughout history. However, the use of herbal supplements during pregnancy adds another degree of complication because the safety and efficacy of many herbs in this context are unknown.

1. Warning: Navigating Uncertainty

Consider a cautionary remark to help you navigate the uncertainties of herbal supplement safety during pregnancy. While certain herbs have well-documented traditional applications and possible advantages, there is a dearth of thorough scientific study on their effects during pregnancy, which raises concerns. To navigate this uncertainty, you must step carefully and seek advice from healthcare professionals.

2. Limited Research: The Pregnancy Study Challenge

Consider the issue of determining the impact of herbal supplements during pregnancy to be inadequate research. Conducting controlled experiments on pregnant women raises ethical concerns, restricting the availability of reliable scientific data. As a result, there are gaps in understanding about the potential hazards and advantages of certain herbs during pregnancy, making informed judgments more difficult.

3. Individual Responses: A One-of-a-Kind Tapestry

Consider individual answers to be a one-of-a-kind tapestry woven by each person's body. Individual responses to herbs, like pregnancy experiences, differ. What one person finds tolerable may cause risk or pain to another. Recognizing the uniqueness of responses emphasizes the significance of personalized caution and consideration while considering herbal supplements.

Herbal Supplements with Pregnancy: Important Factors to Consider

Consider crucial variables that influence the cautious approach needed for your well-being and the best development of your growing baby as you navigate the intricate landscape of herbal supplements during pregnancy.

1. Consultation with a Healthcare Provider: Your Navigation System

Consider a visit with your healthcare professional to be the compass that guides you through the world of herbal supplements. Consult your healthcare provider before introducing any herbs into your routine. Share your goals, talk about your health history, and get advice on the safety of various herbs during pregnancy. Your healthcare professional can provide tailored recommendations depending on your specific circumstances.

2. Potential Risks and Interactions: The Concerns Mosaic

Consider potential dangers and interactions to be a mosaic of problems that may arise from the usage of herbal supplements. Some plants are recognized to be contraindicated during pregnancy, providing concerns of harmful effects or prescription interactions. A prudent strategy entails investigating potential dangers linked with individual herbs and taking into account how they may interact with any drugs you are taking.

3. Dosage and Formulation: Creating a Harmonious Blend

Consider dose and formulation to be the creation of a well-balanced composition for the use of herbal supplements during pregnancy. Herbal supplement potency can vary greatly, and excessive quantities might be dangerous. Select goods with properly labeled dosages and reputed companies that uphold quality standards. Consider herbal formulations that are specifically made for pregnancy, with an emphasis on safety and balance.

4. Traditional Knowledge: A Lighthouse

Consider traditional knowledge to be a guiding light that illuminates the past applications of herbs. While ancient wisdom has been passed down through generations, it must be approached with caution. Some herbs that have been used for centuries may lack scientific confirmation or contain contradictory information about their safety during pregnancy. For a more balanced perspective, combine traditional knowledge with modern caution.

5. A Closer Look at Commonly Used Herbs

Consider regularly used herbs as specific examples that demand cautious attention during pregnancy. While the list of plants to avoid is lengthy, here are a few examples:

Ginger: Ginger, which is commonly used to relieve nausea, is generally considered safe during pregnancy when ingested in moderation.

Excessive doses, on the other hand, may pose hazards, so consult with your healthcare provider.

Peppermint: Peppermint tea, known for its calming effects, is generally considered safe during pregnancy. Peppermint oil in concentrated forms, on the other hand, should be used with caution.

Chamomile: While chamomile tea is commonly used to relax, its safety during pregnancy is debatable. Some studies reveal a possible link to premature labor, therefore use caution, especially in the first trimester.

Echinacea: The safety of echinacea during pregnancy is unknown. It is commonly used for immunological support. There has been limited research, and caution is advised, especially in the absence of clear proof.

St. John's Wort: St. John's Wort, known for its mood-stabilizing qualities, is generally prohibited during pregnancy due to potential hazards to the developing fetus.

Pregnancy and Herbal Supplements: Specific Considerations for Popular Herbs

Consider special precautions and considerations for certain popular herbs as you traverse the terrain of herbal supplements during pregnancy.

1. Ginger (Zingiber officinale): Moderate Nausea Relief

Consider ginger as a therapy for nausea alleviation, with the proviso that it should be used with caution during pregnancy. While ginger is usually regarded safe and may help relieve pregnancy-related nausea, taking too much of it, such as in supplement form, may pose dangers. Before introducing ginger supplements into your routine, consult with your healthcare physician.

2. Peppermint (Mentha piperita): Sensible Soothing

Consider peppermint to be a calming herb with sensitivity throughout pregnancy. When drank in moderation, peppermint tea is generally regarded as safe. However, concentrated forms of peppermint oil should be avoided because they might be toxic, powerful and perhaps harmful. Use caution and get advice from your healthcare provider.

3. Chamomile (Matricaria chamomilla): Caution and Debate

Consider chamomile to be a controversial herb that should be avoided during pregnancy. While chamomile tea is often consumed for relaxation, there is conflicting information about its safety. Some research suggests a possible link to preterm labor. Use chamomile carefully, especially during the first trimester, and consult your healthcare professional.

4. Echinacea (Echinacea purpurea): Uncertainty in Immune Support

Consider echinacea as a plant with immune-boosting potential but uncertainty during pregnancy. There has been little research on the safety of echinacea during pregnancy, so proceed with caution. Consider other immune support techniques and consult with your healthcare physician in the absence of solid data.

5. Hypericum perforatum (St. John's Wort): Mood Stabilization Contradictions

Consider St. John's Wort to be a plant with contradictory effects on mood stability during pregnancy. While this herb is well-known for its mood-stabilizing characteristics, it is typically advised against using it during pregnancy due to potential hazards to the developing fetus. Under the supervision of your healthcare professional, use caution and investigate alternate techniques to mood support.

Holistic Pregnancy: Combining Caution with Individualized Wellness

When it comes to herbal supplements during pregnancy, use a comprehensive strategy that combines caution with individual wellbeing. Recognize that being cautious does not rule out the possible advantages of herbs; rather, it underlines the need of making informed decisions and receiving tailored care.

1. Personalized Wellness: Your One-of-a-Kind Journey

Consider individualized wellness as your personal pregnant journey. What works for one person may not work for another, highlighting the significance of personalized care. Your approach to herbal supplements should be tailored to your health history, preferences, and the advice of your healthcare professional.

2. Whole Foods: Nutrient-Rich Building Blocks

Consider whole foods to be the nutrient-dense foundations that will sustain your pregnancy. While herbal supplements have their place, a well-balanced diet rich in key nutrients from whole foods should be prioritized. Whole foods provide a wide variety of vitamins, minerals, and other valuable components that contribute to your general health and the health of your growing kid.

3. Mind-Body Techniques for Holistic Well-Being

Consider mind-body practices to be contributors to overall well-being throughout pregnancy. Incorporate relaxation and stress-reduction methods into your daily routine, such as meditation, yoga, and deep breathing. These holistic ways can improve your general well-being without the risks linked with some herbal supplements.

4. Hydration and Exercise: Important Elements

Consider hydration and exercise to be essential components of a healthy pregnancy. Staying hydrated and getting regular, pregnancy-appropriate activity help to improve your overall health. These fundamental ingredients strengthen your body's resilience and contribute to a positive pregnant experience.

5. Professional Advice: Making Informed Decisions

Consider professional advice to be the foundation of making informed decisions throughout pregnancy. Your healthcare practitioner is an invaluable resource, providing tailored advice and insights based on their understanding of your medical history. Engage in open discussion, explain your intentions about herbal supplements, and work together to develop a care plan that is in line with your overall health.

Use Caution When Using Herbal Supplements

Navigating the world of herbal supplements during pregnancy is a delicate ballet of caution and consideration. While herbs have a long history in traditional medicine, their safety during pregnancy is still unknown. Approach herbal supplements with skepticism, seek professional advice, and incorporate prudence into your holistic approach for a pregnancy journey that prioritizes your health and the optimal development of your growing kid.

The Role of Medical Advice

Visualize your healthcare provider's advice as a beacon of light on your choice of supplements during pregnancy. Your doctor's expertise, personalized to your specific health profile, provides a complete foundation for making educated decisions that foster your well-being and promote your baby's optimal growth.

1. The Individualized Approach: Advice Tailored to You

Consider your healthcare provider's tailored approach, adjusting suggestions to your specific health history, requirements, and circumstances. Recognizing that each pregnancy is unique, your doctor takes into account aspects such as your medical history, pre-existing problems, dietary habits, and lifestyle to provide individualized supplement advice.

2. Nutritional Foundations: The Importance of a Balanced Diet

Consider your doctor emphasizing the importance of nutrient-rich foundations and a balanced diet throughout pregnancy. While supplements have their place, your doctor emphasizes that entire foods include a wide range of critical nutrients. A well-balanced diet rich in fruits, vegetables, whole grains, lean proteins, and dairy or dairy alternatives is the foundation of a successful pregnancy.

3. Folic Acid: The Building Block of Neural Tube Health

Consider folic acid to be the foundation of neural tube health, with your doctor emphasizing its critical function in preventing neural tube malformations. To ensure the optimal development of your baby's spine and brain throughout the early stages of pregnancy, your healthcare professional advises a prenatal vitamin with the appropriate quantity of folic acid, often 400 micrograms per day.

4. Iron Supplementation: Meeting Rising Demands

Consider iron supplementation to help your body meet the higher needs of pregnancy. Your doctor explains that the growing baby, the placenta, and the increased blood volume all contribute to increased iron requirements. If your doctor identifies or suspects iron deficiency, he or she may offer an iron supplement to avoid anemia and enhance your blood's oxygen-carrying capacity.

5. Calcium: Skeletal Health Protector

Consider calcium to be the defender of skeletal health for both you and your kid, with your doctor emphasizing its importance. Adequate calcium consumption helps your baby's bones and teeth develop while also maintaining your own bone health. Your healthcare professional may suggest a prenatal vitamin with an adequate calcium dosage or dietary changes to meet these needs.

6. Vitamin D Synergy: Improved Calcium Absorption

Consider the interplay of vitamin D and calcium absorption, a potent combo that your doctor emphasizes. While calcium is essential, vitamin D improves absorption, benefiting both you and your baby. Your healthcare professional may advise you to spend time outside for natural sunshine exposure, eat vitamin D-rich foods, or take a supplement if necessary.

7. Omega-3 Fatty Acids: Brain and Vision Nutrition

Consider omega-3 fatty acids to be food for brain and visual growth, with your doctor emphasizing their importance. These essential fats, especially DHA, are critical for your baby's cognitive and visual development. Your doctor may advise you to eat more omega-3-rich foods or to take a DHA-containing prenatal supplement.

8. Iodine: Essential for Thyroid Function

Consider iodine to be vital for thyroid function, which is required for both your metabolism and your baby's cognitive development. To promote normal thyroid function throughout pregnancy, your healthcare professional emphasizes the significance of adequate iodine intake, stressing dietary sources and optional supplementation.

9. Vitamin B12: Support for Red Blood Cells and Nervous System

Consider vitamin B12 to be a supporter of red blood cells and nervous system wellness, with your doctor highlighting its significance. Adequate vitamin B12 consumption prevents anemia and improves nervous system function. If your diet is deficient in B12, your doctor may advise you to take a supplement, especially if you are a vegetarian or vegan.

10. Herbal Supplement Guidance: Navigating Uncertainty

Consider your doctor's advice on herbal supplements as a prudent method to navigating ambiguity. While some herbs have long been used, their safety during pregnancy is unknown. Your healthcare practitioner cautions against the use of specific herbs, emphasizes the significance of discussing them before taking any herbal supplements, and urges openness about any herbal items you may be interested in.

11. Bridging Nutrient Gaps with Tailored Supplement Recommendations

Consider your doctor addressing nutrient deficiencies with individualized supplement suggestions, knowing that everyone's needs differ. Your healthcare professional may propose specific supplements to fill potential gaps in your nutrition for a safe pregnancy based on your health profile and dietary habits.

First Trimester Navigation: Foundational Advice

Your doctor gives basic counsel to set the groundwork for a healthy pregnancy experience as you navigate the first trimester.

1. Prenatal Vitamins for Early Wellness

Consider prenatal vitamins to be the foundation of early wellness throughout the first trimester.

Your doctor advises starting prenatal vitamins early in order to meet crucial nutrient demands, notably folic acid, during the vital early stages of fetal development.

2. Morning Sickness Management: Supplement Adjustment

Consider treating morning sickness with supplement modifications, a more subtle strategy recommended by your doctor. If morning sickness interferes with your capacity to tolerate supplements, your healthcare practitioner may offer special techniques to improve tolerability, such as taking supplements with food or choosing alternate formulations.

3. Tailoring Recommendations Based on Individualized Nutrient Assessments

Consider personalized nutrient evaluations that will help your doctor adjust suggestions to your specific needs. Blood tests may be performed by your healthcare practitioner to analyze nutritional levels, detect any deficiencies, and tailor supplement recommendations based on these results.

Adjustments and Monitoring During the Second Trimester

As you move through the second trimester, your doctor will make modifications and monitor your progress to guarantee your continuing health.

1. Iron Levels: Anemia Risk Assessment

Consider monitoring iron levels during the second trimester to assess the risk of anemia. Periodic blood tests may be performed by your healthcare professional to assess iron levels and, if necessary, modify supplements. This preventive strategy seeks to prevent anemia while also boosting your energy and overall well-being.

2. Optimization of Calcium and Vitamin D: Ensuring Synergy

Consider optimizing calcium and vitamin D levels in order to ensure their synergy for bone health. To ensure optimal amounts of these essential nutrients throughout the second trimester, your doctor may recommend dietary changes, sunlight exposure, or additional treatments.

3. Omega-3 Fatty Acids: Brain Development Support

Consider continuous assistance for omega-3 fatty acids, which are essential for brain growth. To guarantee a regular supply of DHA for your baby's cognitive development, your healthcare professional may examine your dietary consumption of omega-3-rich foods or propose changes to your supplement regimen.

4. Continued Herbal Supplement Guidance: Adapting to Your Journey

Consider ongoing advice on herbal supplements that is tailored to your changing pregnancy adventure. Your healthcare physician will continue to warn you about certain herbs and promotes open discussion about any modifications or additions to your supplement regimen.

As the Third Trimester Approaches: Preparing for Birth

As you enter the third trimester, your doctor will concentrate on delivery preparations and supporting the final phases of fetal development.

1. Iron Supplementation: Meeting Increasing Demand

Consider addressing increasing iron demands during the third trimester, when your baby's demand for iron is at its peak. In preparation for birth, your doctor may reassess your iron status and alter supplements to achieve optimal levels for both you and your baby.

2. Calcium and Vitamin D: Improving Skeletal Health

Consider maintaining skeletal health by paying close attention to calcium and vitamin D.

Because there is still a high demand for these nutrients, your healthcare professional may fine-tune recommendations to support the latter stages of fetal bone growth.

3. Omega-3 Fatty Acids: The Ultimate Brain and Vision Supplement

Consider omega-3 fatty acids as a source of brain and visual assistance during the third trimester. Recognizing the final phases of fetal development before birth, your doctor may reinforce the necessity of a consistent consumption of DHA-rich foods or supplements.

4. Adjustments to Supplements: Reflecting Evolving Needs

Consider supplement changes to match your changing demands in the third trimester. To help you through the last months of pregnancy, your healthcare practitioner monitors changes in your health, reassessing vitamin requirements and changing supplement prescriptions as needed.

Holistic Preparation for Labor and Postpartum

Your doctor gives holistic guidance in the weeks leading up to birth and beyond, including labor preparation and postpartum well-being.

1. Iron Stores: Postpartum Recovery Preparation

Consider your healthcare provider's proactive approach to iron storage for postpartum recovery. Maintaining adequate iron levels not only benefits your well-being throughout labor and delivery, but it also prepares you for postpartum recovery by addressing any blood loss and increasing overall vitality.

2. Ongoing Nutrient Support for Postpartum Wellness

Consider ongoing nutrient support for postpartum wellbeing. Recognizing the continual need of important nutrients during the postpartum period, your doctor may provide advice on maintaining a well-balanced diet and contemplating ongoing supplementation.

3. Postpartum Herbal Supplements: A New Chapter

Consider postpartum herbal supplements as a new phase. Your healthcare professional may revisit herbal supplement discussions, taking into account aspects such as breastfeeding and your overall health. As you negotiate the changing terrain of postpartum care, open communication is crucial.

A Reliable Partner for a Healthy Journey

Your healthcare provider's advice emerges as a trusted collaborator in the vast tapestry of pregnancy, weaving together the intricate threads of nutritional assistance, precautionary advice, and tailored care. Your doctor's insights serve as a compass as you navigate the world of supplements throughout pregnancy, guiding you with expertise, empathy, and a commitment to your well-being and the optimal development of your growing baby. Accept this collaboration, engage in open communication, and proceed with confidence on your pregnancy journey, knowing that you have a determined ally in your healthcare practitioner.

Managing Pregnancy and Existing Health Issues

Pregnancy and pre-existing health conditions are a unique terrain, with your healthcare practitioner functioning as a seasoned guide. As you embark on this journey, their job will become even more important, as they will provide specific recommendations to create a harmonious balance between controlling your health conditions and promoting a healthy pregnancy.

1. Holistic Evaluation: Your Healthcare Provider's Knowledge

Consider your healthcare professional undertaking a comprehensive evaluation of your health, combining their experience with a full awareness of your current situations. This complete review serves as the foundation for tailored counsel, taking into account issues such as chronic conditions, drugs you may be taking, and potential supplement interactions.

2. Individualized Care: Recommendations Tailored to You

Consider customized treatment to be the foundation of your healthcare provider's approach, with supplement suggestions tailored particularly to your health profile. Recognizing that each pregnancy is unique, your doctor considers the complexities of your existing health conditions, ensuring that the supplements recommended correspond with both your health needs and the requirements of a successful pregnancy.

3. A Vital Channel of Communication

Consider open communication to be a crucial conduit throughout this process. Your healthcare provider encourages you to discuss your medical problems, medications, and any concerns you may have. This open exchange of data serves as the foundation for informed decision-making and collaborative care.

Managing Chronic Conditions: Safely Integrating Supplements

As you manage chronic health concerns during pregnancy, your healthcare practitioner will advise you on how to properly use supplements to ensure the best possible support for both you and your baby.

1. Diabetes: Maintaining Blood Sugar Balance

Consider diabetes management throughout pregnancy, when your healthcare professional emphasizes the necessity of blood sugar balance. If you're already on diabetic drugs or insulin, your doctor will look for potential interactions with prenatal vitamins. They may change your supplement routine to prevent interfering with blood sugar management while still ensuring you get the nutrients you need for a healthy pregnancy.

2. Hypertension: Considerations for Sodium and Nutrient Balance

Consider managing hypertension with your healthcare professional focusing on sodium and total nutrient balance. If you're using blood pressure medication, your doctor will consider any sodium content in supplements. They may suggest changes to maintain an ideal nutrient balance, which will benefit both your cardiovascular health and the demands of your growing kid.

3. Thyroid Disorders: Getting Enough Iodine
Consider addressing thyroid issues with your healthcare professional focusing on ensuring enough iodine consumption. Thyroid disorders frequently necessitate unique precautions, particularly when it comes to iodine supplementation. Your doctor carefully assesses your iodine requirements and may change your prenatal supplements to give tailored support for both thyroid function and fetal development.

4. Autoimmune Disorders: Immune Stimulation Without Overstimulation

Consider managing autoimmune illnesses during pregnancy, in which your healthcare professional aims to offer immunological support while avoiding overstimulation. Certain supplements can have an effect on the immune system, and your doctor will look for potential interactions with medications used to treat autoimmune disorders. You navigate a method that promotes your immune health without causing negative side effects together.

Medication Interactions: Protecting Maternal and Fetal Health

Your healthcare practitioner is cautious in protecting maternal and fetal well-being while you manage pregnancy with current health concerns and medications.

1. Evaluating Medication-Supplement Interactions: A Tightrope Walk

Consider your doctor reviewing potential medication-supplement interactions as a fine balance. Some supplements can interfere with drug absorption or efficacy. Your doctor performs a thorough examination, finding any potential conflicts and customizing your supplement plan to complement your medications without interfering with their performance.

2. Vitamin K Considerations in Anticoagulant Medications

Consider controlling anticoagulant drugs and having your healthcare professional handle vitamin K concerns. Anticoagulants may affect vitamin K metabolism, and your doctor will determine whether adjustments are necessary to maintain a delicate balance between promoting blood clotting and preventing excessive bleeding.

3. Antidepressants and Mood Stabilizers: Mood and Nutrient Status Monitoring

Consider navigating pregnancy while taking antidepressants or mood stabilizers, with your healthcare professional keeping track of both your mood and nutritional status. Certain drugs can have an effect on nutritional absorption or utilization. Your doctor carefully evaluates potential interactions and modifies your supplement prescription to support both your mental health and the nutritional requirements of pregnancy.

4. Folate and Vitamin D Considerations in Anticonvulsant Medications

Consider managing anticonvulsant drugs with your healthcare practitioner taking into account the folate and vitamin D consequences. Some anticonvulsants may impact folate metabolism, highlighting the importance of close monitoring and possible changes to your prenatal vitamins. Additionally, your vitamin D status is evaluated to ensure that you and your baby have good skeletal health.

Health-Related Supplement Adjustments: A Dynamic Process

The process of supplement modifications depending on health difficulties is dynamic throughout your pregnant experience, reflecting the changing needs of both you and your baby.

1. Continual Monitoring: Adapting to Changing Needs

Consider regular monitoring to be an important part of adjusting to shifting supplement requirements. Periodic assessments are performed by your healthcare provider, taking into account factors such as changes in health status, medication adjustments, and the advancement of your pregnancy. This continual examination enables you to make timely and focused changes to your supplement program.

2. Nutrient Testing: Personalized Recommendations

Consider nutrient testing to be a tool for customizing suggestions based on your individual nutrient levels. Blood tests may be performed by your doctor to measure essential nutrient levels, guiding supplement modifications depending on your specific needs. This tailored approach guarantees that you get enough necessary nutrients while avoiding excesses.

3. Nutritional Counseling: Dietary and Supplemental Strategies

Consider nutritional advice to be an essential component of integrating dietary and supplementary therapies. Your healthcare physician may work with a certified dietitian to help you optimize your nutritional intake through whole foods as well as supplements. This holistic strategy tries to address specific health issues while also boosting general pregnant well-being.

Expert Guidance Promotes Well-Being

The expert advice from your healthcare practitioner appears as a vital thread in the big tapestry of pregnancy interlaced with existing health conditions. This advice not only guides you through the complexities of supplements and interactions, but it also promotes your overall well-being and the optimal development of your growing kid.

As you continue on this incredible adventure, appreciate the collaborative relationship you have with your healthcare practitioner. Participate in the decision-making process by engaging in open communication, including any changes in your health state or concerns. The advice you receive is not simply about dealing with existing health difficulties; it is a comprehensive approach that spans your complete pregnancy experience, instilling confidence and well-being. You and your healthcare practitioner collaborate to create a maternal health narrative that emphasizes the delicate balance between controlling health issues and encouraging the thriving birth of new life within.

Conclusion

You have launched a profound examination of maternal well-being in the closing pages of your journey through the complexities of pregnancy, supplementation, and the special obstacles posed by existing health concerns. This book has served as a guide, a companion, and a source of understanding, weaving together the threads of science, individualized care, and the unbounded spirit of this life-changing chapter.

Remember, as you close these pages, that the tapestry of pregnancy is as unique as each mother's embrace. With care and deliberation, the importance of diet throughout pregnancy, the role of vitamins and supplements, and the subtle concerns for those navigating current health issues have been emphasized. The importance of healthcare providers' advice, the need of a balanced diet, and the cautious approach to supplements, particularly in the context of herbal medicines, have all been investigated.

You've delved into the complicated dance of sustenance that supports the development of your growing baby in the chapters covering major vitamins and crucial minerals. From Vitamin A to Omega-3 Fatty Acids, the insights into the significance of each nutrient have been offered with the purpose of empowering you to make informed choices that connect with your individual journey.

You've traversed a landscape that requires a delicate balance through the perspective of existing health difficulties. Collaboration with your healthcare provider, concerns for chronic diseases, and the careful integration of supplements with pharmaceuticals have all been identified as critical parts of protecting maternal and fetal well-being.

Imagine this book as a compass guiding you through the stages of pregnancy, providing insights into the changing requirements of both you and your baby as you progress through the trimesters. The narrative has been built to help you as you nurture the marvel of life within, from the fundamental support of prenatal vitamins to the tailored changes based on health circumstances.

Recognize, at the end of this book, that your journey is a constantly unfolding story that is unique to you. The ideas provided here are stepping stones that will help you navigate the complexity of maternal health with knowledge, resilience, and an understanding of the value of holistic well-being. Your healthcare practitioner is not only a guide, but also a partner in this journey, providing expertise and support as you negotiate the unexplored realms of pregnancy.

Carry with you the wisdom learned, the questions answered, and the realization that your well-being is at the heart of the tale as you move beyond these pages. Embrace this changing period with confidence, trust in your body's strength, and rejoice in the deep miracle of life that is happening within you.

May the rest of your pregnancy be full with joy, anticipation, and a deep connection to the magnificent trip you're on. Here's to the next chapter, the arrival of new life, and the continuing of motherhood's wonderful tapestry.

Bonus

Nutritional Meal Plan For Pregnant Women and Expecting Mothers

Quinoa and Chickpeas Power Bowl

Ingredients:

- 1 cup quinoa, cooked
- 1 cup chickpeas cooked (canned or boiled)
- 1 cup chopped spinach
- 1/2 cup halved cherry tomatoes
- 1/2 diced cucumber
- 1/4 cup crumbled feta cheese
-2 tbsp. extra-virgin olive oil
-1 tbsp. balsamic vinegar
1 tablespoon Dijon mustard
- Season with salt and pepper to taste
- Optional garnish: avocado slices

Instructions:

1. Prepare the quinoa and chickpeas as follows:

- Cook the quinoa according to the package directions.
- If using canned chickpeas, rinse and drain them first. If you're boiling them, make sure they're done till soft.

2. Prepare the Bowl:

- Combine cooked quinoa, chickpeas, chopped spinach, cherry tomatoes, cucumber, and crumbled feta cheese in a large mixing basin.

3. Make the dressing:

- Whisk together the olive oil, balsamic vinegar, Dijon mustard, salt, and pepper in a small basin. Season with salt and pepper to taste.

4. Toss and drizzle:

- Dress the quinoa and chickpea combination with the dressing.
- Toss the ingredients gently until evenly coated with the dressing.

5. Garnish and serve:

- Divide the mixture among four serving bowls.
- Garnish with avocado slices, if preferred, for extra creaminess and vitamin richness.

Take your time, taste each bite, and appreciate the nutrient-rich richness in every bite.

This power bowl has protein, fiber, healthy fats, and vitamins, making it a well-balanced and nourishing meal for both you and your growing baby.

This nutrient-dense meal is intended to deliver critical nutrients such as protein, iron, folate, and fiber—all of which are necessary for a healthy pregnancy. Adjust ingredients based on personal preferences and dietary restrictions, and always get specific nutrition advice from your healthcare professional.

Salmon and Quinoa Stuffed Bell Peppers

Ingredients:
- 2 large (any color) bell peppers
- 1 cup quinoa, cooked
- 1 can (6 oz) drained and flaked wild-caught salmon
- 1 cup chopped baby spinach
- 1/2 cup chopped cherry tomatoes
- 1/4 cup coarsely chopped red onion
- 2 teaspoons chopped fresh parsley
1 teaspoon olive oil
-1 tablespoon lemon zest
- 1 tbsp. lemon juice
- 1/2 tsp garlic powder
- Season with salt and pepper to taste
- Optional: grated Parmesan cheese for topping

Instructions:
1. Preheat the oven to 350°F.
- Preheat the oven to 375 degrees Fahrenheit (190 degrees Celsius).

2. Prepare the bell peppers as follows:

- Remove the seeds and membranes from the bell peppers by cutting them in half lengthwise.
- In a baking dish, place the pepper halves.

3. Make the Filling:

- Combine cooked quinoa, flaked salmon, chopped spinach, cherry tomatoes, red onion, and fresh parsley in a large mixing bowl.

4. To make the dressing:

- Whisk together olive oil, lemon zest, lemon juice, garlic powder, salt, and pepper in a small bowl.

5. Toss and combine:

- Dress the quinoa and salmon combination with the dressing.
- Toss until all of the ingredients are evenly coated.

6. Fill the Peppers:

- Fill each half of a bell pepper with the quinoa and salmon mixture.

7. Bake:

- Bake for 25-30 minutes, or until the peppers are cooked, in a preheated oven.

8. Optional garnish:
- For a great finishing touch, sprinkle grated Parmesan cheese over the stuffed peppers during the last 5 minutes of baking.

9. Serve and have fun:
- Warm the filled bell peppers.
- This nutritious recipe contains omega-3 fatty acids from the salmon, protein from both the salmon and the quinoa, and a variety of vitamins and minerals from the vegetables.

Enjoy this delectable and nutritious meal that not only satisfies your taste buds but also supports your and your growing baby's nutritional needs throughout pregnancy.

Tomato-Spinach Sauce with Whole Grain Pasta

Ingredients:
- 2 cups whole grain pasta of choice
- 2 teaspoons olive oil
- 1 finely chopped onion
- 2 minced garlic cloves
- 1 crushed tomato can (14 oz)
1 tablespoon dried oregano
- 1 tsp. dried basil
- Season with salt and pepper to taste
- 2 cups chopped fresh spinach
- Optional garnish: grated Parmesan cheese

Instructions:
1. Prepare the Whole Grain Pasta:
- A big saucepan of salted water should be brought to a boil.
- Cook the whole grain pasta until al dente according to package directions.
- Set aside after draining.

2. To make the Tomato Spinach Sauce, follow these steps:
- Warm the olive oil in a large skillet over medium heat.
- Sauté the finely chopped onion until transparent.

3. Garlic and spices, if using:
- Stir in the minced garlic and cook for 1 minute, or until fragrant.
- Add the dried oregano, dry basil, salt, and pepper to taste. Combine thoroughly.

4. Include Crushed Tomatoes:
- Bring the mixture to a gentle simmer after adding the smashed tomatoes.
- Allow the sauce to simmer for 10-15 minutes to let the flavors mingle and the sauce thicken.

5. Chop the spinach:
- Allow the chopped fresh spinach to wilt into the sauce before stirring it in.

6. Combine the pasta and the sauce:
- Combine the cooked whole grain pasta with the tomato spinach sauce in a skillet.

- Toss the pasta in the sauce and spinach until evenly coated.

7. Seasoning should be adjusted as follows:
- Taste and adjust the seasoning with salt and pepper to your liking.

8. Garnish and serve:
- Individually plate the whole grain spaghetti with tomato and spinach sauce.
- Garnish with grated Parmesan cheese for extra taste.

Enjoy this healthful and savory pasta meal made with whole grains, tomatoes, and spinach.

This nutritious meal has a well-balanced mix of complex carbs, vitamins, and minerals, making it a good choice for both maternal and fetal health. Change the quantities and ingredients to suit your taste.

Lentils and Vegetable Soup

Ingredients:
- 1 cup rinsed and drained dried lentils
- 1 diced onion
- 2 peeled and sliced carrots
- 2 chopped celery stalks
- 3 minced garlic cloves
- 1 can chopped tomatoes (14 oz)
- 6 cups of vegetable stock
- 1 teaspoon cumin powder
- 1 teaspoon coriander powder
1 teaspoon of paprika
- Season with salt and pepper to taste
- 2 cups chopped kale or spinach
- Optional: fresh lemon wedges for serving

Instructions:
1. Lentils should be prepared as follows:
- Under cold water, rinse and drain the dried lentils.

2. Vegetables Sauté:
- Warm a little olive oil in a big pot over medium heat.

- Mix in the diced onions, carrots, and celery. Cook until the vegetables soften, about 5 minutes.

3. Garlic and spices, if using:

- Stir in the minced garlic and cook for another minute, or until fragrant.
- Mix in the cumin, coriander, paprika, salt, and pepper. Mix thoroughly to coat the vegetables with the spices.

4. Include Lentils and Tomatoes:

- Pour in the washed lentils and stir to combine.
- Mix in the diced tomatoes (with their juice).

5. Add the vegetable broth:

- Pour in the vegetable broth, making sure the lentils are completely submerged.

6. Simmer:

- Bring the soup to a boil, then lower to a low heat, cover, and leave to cook for 25-30 minutes, or until the lentils are cooked.

7. Leafy greens should be added:

- Cook for an additional 5 minutes, or until the greens are wilted, after adding the chopped kale or spinach.

8. Seasoning should be adjusted as follows:

- Taste the soup and adjust the seasoning with salt and pepper to your liking.

9. Serve:

- Pour the lentil and vegetable soup into serving dishes.
- Serve with a wedge of fresh lemon, if desired, for a blast of citrus flavor.

Enjoy this filling and healthy lentil and vegetable soup, which is high in protein, fiber, and important vitamins.

Feel free to change the vegetables or seasonings to your liking. This soup is not only tasty but also high in plant-based protein and other minerals.

Chia Seed Pudding with Mango

Ingredients:
1 tablespoon chia seeds
1 cup almond milk (or other milk of choice)
1 tbsp honey or maple syrup (optional, for added sweetness)
a half teaspoon of vanilla extract
1 diced ripe mango
Garnish with fresh mint leaves (optional).

Instructions:
Chia Seeds and Almond Milk should be combined:
- Combine the chia seeds, almond milk, honey (if using), and vanilla essence in a mixing dish.
- Whisk together the ingredients until completely incorporated.

Allow it to Set:
- Refrigerate the chia seed mixture for at least 4 hours, or better overnight.

- The chia seeds will absorb the liquid and form a pudding-like consistency during this time.

Before serving, give the following a good stir:

- To ensure a uniform texture, give the chia seed pudding a quick stir before serving.

Assemble the following with Mango:

- Cut the ripe mango into bite-sized chunks.
- Layer the chia seed pudding and diced mango in serving glasses or bowls.

Optional garnish:

- For enhanced freshness and visual appeal, garnish with fresh mint leaves.

Serve:

- Immediately serve the Chia Seed Pudding with Mango.

Enjoy this delectable and healthy dessert or brunch alternative.

This Chia Seed Pudding with Mango is not only tasty but also high in fiber, omega-3 fatty acids, and vitamins. Feel free to adjust the sweetness and toppings to suit your taste.

Lean Turkey and Vegetable Stir Fry

Ingredients:
1 pound ground turkey
2 tbsp (low-sodium) soy sauce
1 teaspoon oyster sauce
1 tbsp sesame seed oil
2 minced garlic cloves
1 tablespoon grated fresh ginger
2 cups florets broccoli
1 finely sliced bell pepper
1 julienned carrot
1 cup trimmed snap peas
2 sliced green onions
1 tsp cornstarch (optional for thickening)
Brown rice, cooked and ready to serve

Instructions:
Prepare the turkey as follows:
- Heat a little oil in a big skillet or wok over medium-high heat.

- Cook until the lean ground turkey is browned, breaking it up with a spatula.

Make the Sauce:
- Combine soy sauce, oyster sauce, and sesame oil in a small bowl.

Add Aromatics:
- Make a space in the center of the skillet by pushing the browned turkey to the side.
- Sauté the minced garlic and grated ginger in the middle until aromatic.

Mix with Vegetables:
- In the skillet, combine the broccoli, bell pepper, carrot, and snap peas.
- Stir-fry the veggies with the turkey for 3-4 minutes, or until soft but still crisp.

Include the following sauce:
- Serve the turkey and veggies with the sauce.
- Toss everything together in the sauce until fully coated.

Optional thickening:
- If you want a thicker sauce, make a slurry with 1 tablespoon cornstarch and a little

water. Stir it into the stir-fry until the sauce thickens.

Add the green onions:

* Stir in the sliced green onions for another minute.

Serve:

* Serve the stir-fry of lean turkey and vegetables over cooked brown rice.

As a healthful and filling meal, serve this tasty and protein-packed stir-fry.

Feel free to modify the vegetables or seasoning to your desire. This dish contains a good combination of lean protein and colorful vegetables, making it a nutritious choice for a quick and tasty meal.

Eggs and Spinach Breakfast Wrap

Ingredients:
two huge eggs
1 cup spinach leaves, fresh
1 whole-wheat tortilla
Season with salt and pepper to taste.
Salsa, avocado slices, and shredded cheese are optional garnishes.

Instructions:
Sauté the spinach:
- Warm a small amount of olive oil in a nonstick skillet over medium heat.
- Sauté fresh spinach leaves until wilted. Place aside.

Eggs Scrambled:
- Crack two eggs into a bowl and whisk them in the same skillet.
- Over medium heat, pour the whisked eggs into the skillet.

Season the eggs as follows:

- Season the eggs to taste with salt and pepper.
- Allow the eggs to sit for a few seconds before gently scrambling them with a spatula until fully done.

Tortilla Soup:

- Warm the whole-grain tortilla in the skillet for a few seconds.

Put the Wrap Together:

- Place the hot tortilla on a platter.
- Scramble the eggs in the center of the tortilla.

Sauté the spinach:

- Place the scrambled eggs on top of the sautéed spinach.

Optional Extras:

- If desired, garnish with salsa, avocado slices, or shredded cheese.

To sum it up:

- Fold in the tortilla's sides and roll it up to make a wrap.

Serve:

- Immediately serve the egg and spinach breakfast sandwich.

Enjoy this quick and nutritious meal that combines egg protein with spinach deliciousness.

Feel free to add your favorite toppings or extra vegetables to the wrap. This meal is not only tasty, but it is also high in protein and important nutrients to get your day started.

Greek Yogurt Parfait with Berries and Nuts

Ingredients:
1 cup plain Greek yogurt
1 granola cup
1/2 cup berries (strawberries, blueberries, and raspberries)
1 tbsp honey or maple syrup (optional, for added sweetness)
2 tbsp. chopped nuts (almonds, walnuts, or other nuts of your choosing)

Instructions:
Greek Yogurt Layer:
- Begin by layering Greek yogurt in a glass or a bowl.

Granola can be added:
- Sprinkle granola on top of the Greek yogurt.

Berries on top:
- On top of the granola, put a layer of mixed berries.

Layers that should be repeated:

- Repeat the layers by adding more Greek yogurt, granola, and berries until the appropriate amount is reached.

Drizzle with honey if desired:

- Drizzle honey or maple syrup over the parfait for added sweetness.

Chopped Nuts (optional):

- Finish by putting chopped nuts on top of the parfait.

Serve:

- Serve the Greek Yogurt Parfait right away.

Enjoy this tasty and nutritious parfait, which contains protein, fiber, vitamins, and healthy fats.

Feel free to add your favorite fruits, nuts, or other toppings to the parfait. This adaptable and filling breakfast or snack is not only delicious but also a terrific way to include a variety of nutrients into your diet.

Sweet Potatoes and Chickpeas Curry

Ingredients:
2 medium-sized peeled and sliced sweet potatoes
1 can (15 oz) washed and drained chickpeas
1 finely chopped onion
2 minced garlic cloves
1 tablespoon grated ginger
1 can chopped tomatoes (14 oz)
1 coconut milk can (14 oz)
two tbsp curry powder
1 teaspoon cumin powder
1 teaspoon coriander powder
a half teaspoon turmeric
1/4 teaspoon cayenne pepper (to taste)
Season with salt and pepper to taste.
2 tbsp oil for cooking
Garnish with fresh cilantro
Serve with cooked rice

Instructions:

Onion, garlic, and ginger sauté:
- Heat the cooking oil in a big pot or deep pan over medium heat.
- Sauté the finely chopped onion until softened.
- Sauté the minced garlic and grated ginger for another minute, or until fragrant.

Spices to taste:
- Combine curry powder, ground cumin, ground coriander, turmeric, cayenne pepper, salt, and pepper in a mixing bowl.
- Allow the spices to roast for approximately a minute in the onion mixture.

Add sweet potatoes and chickpeas:
- To the pot, add diced sweet potatoes and drained chickpeas.
- Stir in the spice mixture to coat the sweet potatoes and chickpeas.

Combine:
- Add the diced tomatoes (with juice) and coconut milk.
- Bring the mixture to a low heat.

Cook until the sweet potatoes are tender:

- Allow the curry to boil for 20-25 minutes, or until the sweet potatoes are cooked.
- Seasoning should be adjusted as follows:
- If required, taste the curry and adjust the seasoning.

Serve with rice:

- Over cooked rice, serve the sweet potato and chickpea curry.

Garnish and Serve:

- Before serving, garnish with fresh cilantro.
- Enjoy this warm and fragrant sweet potato and chickpea curry.

You can tweak the spice levels and customize the curry by adding extra vegetables if desired. This dish is a tasty and healthful way to include sweet potatoes and chickpeas in your diet.

Stir-Fry Vegetables with Tofu

Ingredients:
1 firm tofu block, pressed and cubed
2 tbsp (low-sodium) soy sauce
1 teaspoon hoisin sauce
1 tbsp sesame seed oil
1 tbsp. vegetable oil
2 minced garlic cloves
1 tablespoon grated fresh ginger
1 finely sliced bell pepper
1 julienned carrot
1 cup florets broccoli
1 cup trimmed snap peas
2 sliced green onions
Optional: 1 tablespoon sesame seeds
Serve with cooked brown rice or noodles.

Instructions:
Tofu Pressed and Cubed:
- Place the tofu between paper towels and gently press it to remove any excess water.
- Tofu should be cut into cubes.

Marinate the tofu:

- Toss cubed tofu with soy sauce, hoisin sauce, and sesame oil in a mixing dish.
- Allow at least 15-20 minutes for the tofu to marinade.

Sauté the tofu:

- Heat the vegetable oil in a large skillet or wok over medium-high heat.
- Cook until the marinated tofu cubes are golden brown on all sides.
- Set the tofu aside after removing it from the skillet.

Vegetable Stir-Fry:

- If necessary, add a little additional oil to the same skillet.
- Sauté the minced garlic and grated ginger for a minute, or until fragrant.
- Add the bell pepper, carrot, broccoli florets, and snap peas.
- Cook until the vegetables are tender-crisp.

Tofu and vegetables should be combined:

- Return the sautéed tofu to the skillet with the vegetables.
- Toss everything together until everything is fully integrated.

Finishing and garnishing:
- Sprinkle the stir-fry with chopped green onions and sesame seeds (if using).
- Toss one more to spread the ingredients evenly.

Serve:
- Serve the tofu-vegetable stir-fry over cooked brown rice or noodles.

Enjoy this tasty and healthy vegetable stir-fry with tofu.

Feel free to add your favorite vegetables or sauce to the stir-fry. This dish is high in plant-based protein and has a range of bright vegetables.